❧ The Many Faces Of Cancer ❧

Their True Stories

By: Lori Fundal Pilatan

Table of Contents

All medical terms used in this book are taken from: American Cancer Society, Canadian Cancer Society, PSW text book, googles, Mayo Clinic and Wikipedia 211

Introduction

There are so many people who have been touched by cancer. Personally, my friends, my cousins, my adopted mother, my adopted sister and her sister, my niece, my nephew's wife and recently my sister, they had all been touched by cancer. Some had survived, but not all had been lucky. I am a primary caregiver of five of those I had mentioned. I did not only witness their suffering, but I was also part of their journey living life with cancer. I believe cancer is much harder on the loved ones, especially on the primary caregiver than it is on those who have been diagnosed with cancer.

Cancer is a lifetime journey; from enduring cancer diagnosis and subsequent treatment can be emotionally and physically draining. Some people anticipate that once they successfully finish cancer treatment, their lives will resume as normal. However, many find that lingering physical side effects create new issues and concerns that they might not have anticipated.

The individual stories that you will read about in this book are examples of touching raw emotion that exacerbates when they've been told they had cancer.

It tells a heart wrenching story about their struggles living with cancer. It tells about the inspirational story of resilience, courage, strength and hope in the face of overwhelming odds. It explores and shares the author's personal experience caring for her loved ones at home and hospital, revealing with utter honesty, and catching humor in moments of utter darkness and light, of intense pain and blissful but precarious relief. The many faces of cancer: their true story, captures the trauma of a cancer diagnosis, treatment, after treatment and their journey to survive the disease.

As a primary caregiver, the author describes in this book her role caring for her loved ones diagnosed with cancer. Caring for someone with cancer isn't easy. It often involves taking many responsibilities. It can go on for a long time – many months or years. It's not something you expect or plan ahead for. The responsibility can be overwhelming, stressful, and extremely challenging but it can also be very rewarding in knowing that you were there for your loved ones in their difficult journey living with cancer.

This book will also encourage that you can be a caregiver for someone even if you don't live very close to you. My sister in the Philippines who had been diagnosed with cancer, our distance didn't deter my involvement with her care. I stay involved with decisions about her care and treatment by using conference calls through social media; Facebook [messenger]. In which I am grateful because social media helped me keep in touch with my sister by using messenger video call feature. A simple phone call can make a whole lot of difference to someone who has been diagnosed with cancer.

My wish in writing this book is that somehow I may be able to put a face to every suffering, struggles and journey of those who courageously fought to survive this evil disease. Likewise, I would also like to share the difficult tasks and role of being a primary caregiver both emotionally and psychologically. My other reason for writing this book is to encourage people that regardless of a difficult journey ahead is to never lose hope – keep a positive outlook even in the midst of darkness. Keep smiling and enjoy life every moment. The most important thing, never let go of your loved ones hand – keep holding their hand until the end.

Dedication

I dedicate this book to honor the courageous, inspirational, valor of all people that had been touched by cancer across the globe, especially those who are in this book. Their journey and struggle to fight cancer to survive is overwhelmingly uplifting and touching. Unfortunately, some of them did not make it, although some have survived and picked up the pieces of their life before cancer.

To my beloved niece, Neneng Sinya who was diagnosed of Acute Myelogenous Leukemia, who died less than two [2] months after she was diagnosed at the age of thirteen [13] years old. It's been over forty years ago, but your memory is still vivid and Crystal clear in my mind how you fought the cancer with courage and determination until the end.

Nana Carling, who was diagnosed with Ovarian cancer at a later stage, against all odds survived the cancer and lived for another three years, after having been told that she had only 2-4 months to live.

To Lita, who was diagnosed with Invasive breast cancer with HER2 positive. I witnessed how bravely you fought cancer. Your faith in God and your determination to live helped you defeat this horrible disease. It's been twelve years since you've been first diagnosed, you did not allow cancer to define you, rather you live your life appreciating the second chance of life God has given you.

To Libeth, diagnosed with Colon cancer. Despite not understanding the full gravity of your illness, you survived the disease.

To Neil, who was diagnosed with Diffuse Large B-Cell Lymphoma [DLBCL] whom I briefly Knew, but admire your determination and courage to survive, but sadly died less than five months after you were diagnosed. A young man with dreams and hope for a brighter future, but cancer snatched your life too early.

To Len, who was diagnosed with Gastrointestinal Stromal Tumor [GIST], your humor and determination helped you survive the disease.

To My cousin, Monina Pascual Estandarte, who was diagnosed with breast cancer. You survived the first year of your treatment and my wish and hope for you that you would become a statistic of those cancer "Alivers", survivors.

To Taciana Sta. Barbara de Otoy, who was diagnosed with cervical cancer. Despite your pain and suffering you never falter in your faith in God. Now, you are at the arm of your creator. No more pain and suffering but joy and peace.

To my beloved sister, Neneng Herminia who was diagnosed with Laryngeal [throat] cancer. I am so appreciative of the social media [FB] because despite our thousand miles distance I was able to talk to you every day. I witnessed how valiantly you fought so hard to survive for your family, especially for your grandchildren's [MC, UK, and Jayden], unfortunately, you died just a little over a year after you had been diagnosed. You may be gone but you will be forever in my heart.

Last but not the least, to all families who bravely stood behind your loved ones in their worst, holding their hands, a pillar of support, encouraging and loving them. This book is also for all of you.

Acknowledgement

Rosalinda Solidarios Palmares, MD, MMEM, FPCP

Master in Management, Major in Educational Management

Former Associate Dean, Iloilo Doctors' College of Medicine

Fellow, Philippines College of Physicians

Secretary, Philippine College of Occupational Medicine, Iloilo – Panay Chapter

I am immensely grateful for editing the medical terms and medical procedures used in this book.

Rosette Andrea Marie S. Palmares, RMT, MD, FPCP

Registered Medical Technologist

Fellow, Philippine College of Physicians

Trained in adult Infectious Diseases at Research Institute for Tropical Medicine

Likewise grateful for editing the medical terms, and medical procedures used in this book.

Len Phillips: Retired Teacher and Editor

Thank you for editing this book.

Jun Estorque: Information Technology [IT]

Thank you for putting the book cover together and getting the book ready for publication.

Ivy Marie Barcelona Pilatan: Medical Student

Thank you for helping me with this book.

To all those who were diagnosed with cancer, thank you for letting me tell your stories.

I would like also to extend my gratitude to all family members who allowed me to share their experienced taking care of their loved ones as the journeyed living with cancer.

Chapter 1

What is cancer?

Cancer is a disease in which some of the body's cells grow uncontrollably and spread to other parts of the body. Cancer affects 1 in 4 people in the world. In most likelihood, you or someone you know has been affected by cancer.

How cancer begins

Cells are the basic units that make up the human body. Cells grow and divide to make new cells as the body needs them.

Cancer begins when genetic changes interfere with this orderly process. Cells start to grow uncontrollably. These cells may form a mass or lump called a tumor. A tumor can be cancerous or benign. A cancerous tumor is malignant and can grow and spread to other body parts. A benign tumor means the tumor can grow but is not cancerous or will not spread.

Cancer can start almost everywhere in the human body. You are made up of trillions of cells that over your lifetime normally grow and divide as needed. Normally, human cells grow and multiply [through a process called cell division] to form new cells as the body needs them. When cells grow old or become damaged, they die, and new cells take their place. Cancer starts when something goes wrong in this process and your cells keep making new cells and the old or abnormal ones don't die when they should. Cancer cells can crowd out normal cells as they grow out of control. This makes it hard for your body to work the way it should.

Sometimes this orderly process breaks down, and abnormal or damaged cells grow and multiply when they shouldn't. These cells may form tumors, which are lumps of tissue. Tumor can be cancerous or not cancerous [benign].

Cancerous tumors spread into, or invade, nearby tissues and can travel to distant places in the body which become malignant tumors. Many cancers form solid tumors, but cancers of the blood, such as leukemias, generally do not.

Benign tumors do not spread into, or invade, nearby tissues. When removed, benign tumors usually don't go back, whereas cancerous tumors sometimes do. Benign tumors can sometimes be quite large, however. Some can be causing serious symptoms or be life-threatening, such as a benign tumor in the brain.

For many people, cancer can be treated successfully. In fact, more people than ever before lead a full life after cancer treatment. Four out of nine people close to me in this book, including my loved ones of whom five of them, I was a primary caregiver survived the cancer and lived a productive life.

Cancer is more than just one disease

There are many types of cancer: Cancer can develop anywhere in the body and is named for the part of the body where it started. For instance, breast cancer that starts in the breast is called breast cancer even if it spreads [metastasizes] to other parts of the body.

There are two main categories of cancer:

- **Hematologic [blood] cancers** are cancers of the blood cells, including leukemia, lymphoma, and multiple myeloma.
- **Solid tumor cancers** are cancers of any of the other body organs or tissues. The most common solid tumors are breast, prostate, lung and colorectal cancers.

These cancers are alike in some ways, but can be different in the way they grow, spread, and respond to treatment. Some cancers grow and spread fast. Others grow more slowly. Some are more likely to spread to other parts of the body. Others tend to stay where they started.

Some types of cancer are best treated with surgery; others respond better to drugs such as chemotherapy. Often 2 or more treatments are used to get the best result.

What is a tumor?

- A tumor is a lump or growth. Some lumps are cancerous, but many are not.
- Lumps that are not cancer are called **benign**
- Lumps that are cancer are called **malignant**

What makes cancer different is that it can spread to other parts of the body while benign tumors do not. Cancer cells can break away from the site where the cancer started. These cells can travel to other parts of the body and end up in the lymph nodes or other body organs causing problems with normal functions.

What causes cancer?

Cancer cells develop because of multiple changes in their genes. These changes can have many possible causes. Lifestyle habits, genes you get from your parents, and being exposed to cancer-causing agents in the environment can all play a role. Many have no obvious cause.

Some types of cancers do not form tumors. These include leukemia, most types of lymphoma, and myeloma.

Types of cancer

Medical experts, or doctors divide cancer into types based on where it started. Four main types of cancers are:

. **Carcinomas.** A carcinoma begins in the skin or the tissue that covers the surface of internal organs and glands. Carcinomas are the most common type of cancer. They are formed by **epithelial** cells, which are the cells that cover the inside and outside surfaces of the body. There are many types of epithelial cells, which often have columns – like shapes when viewed under the microscope.

Carcinomas that begin in different epithelial cells types have specific names:

Adenocarcinoma. Is a cancer that forms in epithelial cells that produce fluids or muscles. Tissues with this type of epithelial cell are sometimes called glandular tissues. Most cancers of the breast, colon, and prostate are this type.

Basal cell adenocarcinoma. Is a cancer that begins in the lower or basal [base] layer of the epidermis, which is a person's outer layer of skin.

Squamous cell carcinoma. Is a cancer that forms in squamous cells, which are epithelial cells that lie just beneath the outer surface of the skin. Squamous cells also line many other organs, including the stomach, intestine, lungs, bladder, and kidney. Squamous cells look flat, like fish scales, when viewed under the microscope. Squamous cell carcinoma is sometimes called **epidermoid** carcinoma.

Transitional cell carcinoma. Is a cancer that forms in a type epithelial tissue called **transitional epithelium,** or **urothelium.** This tissue, which is made up of many layers of epithelial cells that can get bigger and smaller, is found in the lining of the bladder, uterus, and part of the kidneys [renal pelvis], and a few other organs. Some cancers of the bladder, ureters, and kidney are transitional cell carcinoma.

Sarcomas. A sarcoma begins in the tissues that support and connect the body. A sarcoma can develop in fat, muscles, nerves, tendons, joints, blood vessels, lymph vessels, cartilage, or bone.

Leukemias. Leukemia is cancer of the blood. Leukemia begins when healthy blood cells change and grow uncontrollably. Cancer that begins in the blood – forming tissue of the bone marrow are called leukemias. These cancers do not form solid tumors. Instead, large numbers of abnormal white blood cells [leukemia cells and leukemic blast cells] build up in the blood and bone marrow, crowding out normal blood cells. The low level of normal blood cells can make it harder for the body to get oxygen to its tissues, control bleeding, or fight infections. The main types of leukemia are: **lymphocytic leukemia, chronic lymphocytic leukemia, acute myeloid leukemia**, and **chronic myeloid leukemia**.

Lymphomas. Lymphoma is a cancer that begins in the lymphatic system. The lymphatic system is a network of vessels and glands that help fight infection. There are 2 types of lymphomas: **Hodgkin lymphoma** and **non-Hodgkin lymphoma**.

Other types of cancer: According to the study, there are more than 200 types of cancer, and related hereditary syndromes. Every type of cancer has their own characteristics and affects their victims differently. There are many types of cancer treatment. The types of treatment that you receive will depend on the type of cancer you have and how advanced it is. Why are different cancers treated differently? Because according to the study of oncologists cancer cells can be so different, what kills one type of cell might not do anything to another. The best overall treatment involves getting the best out of each specialty.

What is the cancer stage?

When the cancer is found, tests are done to see how big the cancer is and whether it has spread from where it started.

A lower stage [such as a stage 1 or 2] means that the cancer has not spread very much. A higher number [such as a stage 3 or 4] means it has spread more. Stage 4 is the highest stage.

As a cancerous tumor grows, the bloodstream or lymphatic system may carry cancer cells to other parts of the body. During this process, the cancer cells grow and may develop.

Diagnosing: How do doctors diagnose Cancer?

Often, a diagnosis begins when a person visits a doctor about an unusual symptom. The doctor will then ask about the medical history and perform a physical examination. This may also include the personal, social, and family history. After which, the doctor will request for various tests to support the diagnosis of these signs and symptoms.

But many people with cancer have no symptoms. For these people, cancer is diagnosed during a medical test for another issue or condition.

Sometimes a doctor finds cancer after a screening test in an otherwise healthy person.

Health care providers begin a cancer diagnosis by doing a comprehensive physical examination. They'll ask you to describe your symptoms. They may ask about your family history.

They may also do the following tests:

- Blood test
- Imaging
- Biopsies

Blood tests

Blood test for cancer may include:

- **Complete blood count [CBC]**: It measures and counts your red and white blood cells.

- **tumor markers**: Tumor markers are substances that cancer cells release or that your normal cells release in response to cancer cells.
- **blood protein tests**: Health care providers use a process called electrophoresis to measure immunoglobulins. Your immune system reacts to certain cancers by releasing immunoglobulins.
- **Circulating tumor cell tests**:

Cancerous tumors may shed cells. Tracking tumor cells helps healthcare providers monitor cancer activity.

Imaging tests

Imaging tests may include:

- **Computed tomography [CT] scan**:

CT scans check for cancerous tumors' location and impact on your organs and bones.

- **X -rays**: X-rays use safe amounts of radiation to create images of your bones and soft tissues.
- **Position emission test [PET] scan**: Pet scans produce images of your organs and tissues at work. Healthcare providers may use this test to detect early signs of cancer.
- **Ultrasound**: An ultrasound uses high- intensity sound waves that show structures inside of your body.
- **Magnetic resonance imaging [MRI]**: MRIs use a large magnet, radio waves and a computer to create images of your organs and other structures inside of your body.

- **Iodine meta-iodobenzylguanidine [MIGB]**: This nuclear imaging test helps detect cancer, including carcinoid tumors and neuroblastoma.

Biopsies

A biopsy is a procedure healthcare provider do obtain cells, tissues, fluid or growths that they'll examine under a microscope. There are several kinds of biopsies:

- **Needle biopsy**: this test may be called a fine needle aspiration or fine needle biopsy. Healthcare providers use a thin hollow needle and syringe to extract cells, fluid or tissue from suspicious lumps. Needle biopsies are often done to help diagnose breast cancer, thyroid cancer or cancer in your lymph nodes.
- **Skin biopsy**: Healthcare providers remove a small sample of your skin to diagnose skin cancer.
- **Bone marrow biopsy**: Healthcare providers remove a small sample of bone marrow so they can test the sample for signs of the disease, including cancer in your bone.
- **Endoscopic or laparoscopic biopsy**.
- These biopsies use an endoscope or laparoscope to see the inside of your body. With Laparoscopy, a small cut is made in your skin and an instrument is inserted. An endoscopy on the other hand, uses a thin, flexible tube with camera on the tip inserted in a patient's orifice, along with a cutting tool to obtain samples.
- **Excisional or incisional biopsy**: For these open biopsies, a surgeon cuts into your body and either the entire tumor is removed

[excisional biopsy] or part of the tumor is removed [incisional biopsy] to test or treat it.

- **Perioperative biopsy**: This test may be called a frozen section biopsy. This biopsy is done while a surgeon is doing an operation for a related or unrelated reason. Your tissue will be removed and tested right away. Results will come in during the procedure, so if you need treatment, it can start immediately.

Genetic testing

Cancer may happen when a single gene mutates or several genes that work together to mutate. Researchers have identified more than 400 genes associated with cancer development. People who inherit these genes from their biological parents may have an increased risk of developing cancer. Healthcare providers may recommend genetic testing for cancer if you have an inherited form of cancer. They may also do genetic testing to do therapy that targets specific cancer genes. They use test results to develop a diagnosis. They'll assign a number or stage to your diagnosis. The higher the number, the more cancer has spread.

How is the cancer stage determined?

Healthcare providers use cancer staging systems to plan treatment and develop a prognosis or expected outcome. TNM is the most widely used cancer staging. T stands for primary tumor. N stands for lymph nodes and indicates whether a tumor has spread to your lymph nodes. M stands for metastasis, when cancer spreads to other organ.

What are the four stages of cancer?

Most cancers have four stages. The specific stage is determined by a few different factors, including the tumor's size and location:

- **Stage 1**: The cancer is localized to a small area and hasn't spread to lymph nodes or other tissues.
- **Stage 2**: The cancer has grown, but it hasn't spread.
- **Stage 3**: The cancer has grown larger and has possibly spread to lymph nodes or other tissues.
- **Stage 4**: The cancer has spread to other organs or areas of your body. This stage is also referred to as **metastasis** or advanced cancer.

What is metastatic Cancer?

Metastatic cancer occurs when cancer cells break off from the original tumor, enter your bloodstream or lymph system and spread to other areas of your body. Most metastatic cancers are manageable, but not curable. Treatment can ease your symptoms, slow cancer growth and improve your quality of life.

How do healthcare providers treat cancer?

Healthcare providers may use several different treatments, sometimes combining treatments based on your situation, or how far the cancer spread.

Common cancer treatments include:

- **Chemotherapy**: Chemotherapy is one of the most common cancer treatments. It uses powerful drugs to destroy cancer cells. You may receive chemotherapy in pill form or intravenously [through a needle into a vein]. In some cases, providers may be able to direct chemotherapy to the specific area affected.
- **Radiation therapy**: This treatment kills cancer cells with high doses of radiation. Your healthcare provider may combine radiation therapy and chemotherapy.
- **Surgery**: Cancerous tumors that haven't spread or that may need debulking may be removed with surgery. Your healthcare provider may recommend therapy. This treatment combines surgery, with chemotherapy or radiation to shrink a tumor before surgery or kill cancer cells that may remain after surgery.
- **Hormone therapy**: Sometimes, providers prescribe hormones that block other cancer-causing hormones. For example, men who have prostate cancer might receive hormones to keep testosterone [which contributes to prostate cancer] lower than usual.
- **Biological response modifier therapy**: Immunotherapy is a type of biological therapy that engages your immune system to fight the cancer cells. Example are Monoclonal antibodies and vaccines.
- **Targeted therapy for cancer**: Targeted therapy is a cancer treatment that targets the genetic changes or mutations that turn healthy cells into cancer cells.

- **Bone marrow transplant**: Also called stem cell transplantation, this treatment replaces damaged stem cells with healthy ones. Autologous transplantation uses your supply of healthy stem cells. **Allogeneic transplantation** uses stem cells donated by another person.

What are the side effects?

Cancer treatments have been improving for decades. Researchers are not only developing treatments that are more effective, but they are also highly focused on reducing their side effects.

Side effects are problem that affects your healthy tissue and organs as a result of cancer treatment. It can vary from person to person and from treatment to treatment. People receiving the same treatment may experience varied side effects. Some experience side effects that arise during treatment and improve over time, which is the most common scenario.

But some people experience severe side effects that last for months or even years after treatment is completed.

Everybody is different, but there are common side effects due to treatment.

What are the most common side effects of treatment?

Pain. The term "pain" describes a broad category of types of symptoms and it is common to all cancers and cancer treatments. Pain can drastically interfere with your quality of life by making it difficult or impossible to eat, sleep, socialize and do your day-to-day routines. It is important to understand and know that your pain can be treated. Treatment options include pain medication and other therapies recommended by your oncologist or your health team providers.

Example: Five of my loved ones who had been diagnosed with cancer experienced pain. Although some experienced more pain than others.

- **Fatigue**. Cancer - related fatigue [CRF] is a severe form of fatigue often described by people with cancer as an overwhelming tiredness, exhaustion, and weakness that doesn't go away with sleep and rest. Fatigue is perhaps the most common and distressing symptom of cancer treatment and is especially common as a result of chemotherapy.

Example: all the people diagnosed with cancer in this book experienced fatigue and insomnia – they all had difficulty sleeping and at some point the treatment had to be stopped because the red blood cells reached an alarming level; very low.

- **Anemia**. Anemia develops when there are insufficient red blood cells to carry oxygen throughout the body. This can cause dizziness, weakness and increased heart rate. Treatments that can cause anemia include chemotherapy, radiation therapy, and some immunotherapies. This happens because these treatments can inadvertently destroy healthy red blood cells in the process of killing cancer cells.

Example: Three out of five of my loved ones who had been diagnosed with cancer suffered from anemia – lower red blood cells. At some point the treatment had to be canceled or delayed because the red blood cells reached an alarming level that is dangerous to proceeds.

- **Hair, skin, and nail problems**. Radiation therapy can bring hair loss to the part of the body receiving radiation, while chemotherapy can lead to loss of hair on the head and other parts of the body. Different chemotherapy drugs can cause different types of hair loss, or no hair loss at all. Hair loss usually happens within two weeks of treatment, getting worse over the first month or two of ongoing treatment. Regrowth can begin while treatment is still happening, or within one to three months after it is done. Skin – related side effects of chemotherapy and radiation therapy can include dryness, itchiness, redness, and swelling. You should be careful exposing yourself in the sun while receiving treatment because you may be more susceptible to sunburn. You may also experience changes in your nails, like darkening, yellowing, or cracking of the nails and/ or cuticles.

Example: not everybody that had chemotherapy losses their hair. My adopted sister and adopted mother both lost their hair. Whereas, three of them, chemotherapy had no effects on their hair. Although they all experienced other symptoms – skin and nail problems.

- **Mouth problem**. Mouth problems are common with many types of cancer treatments. Anticancer drugs and radiation to the head and neck can damage your salivary glands and tissues in the mouth, throat, and lips. This can cause difficulty swallowing, changes in taste, dry mouth, infections in the mouth, mouth sores, tooth decay and sensitivity to hot and cold food.

Example: all of my loved ones were diagnosed with cancer, they all suffered mouth problems, especially dried mouth and sores.

- **Nausea and vomiting**. Immunotherapy, radiation therapy to the abdomen, and chemotherapy [with results varying by the type of drug and its dose] are all known to cause nausea and vomiting in people receiving cancer treatment. Nausea and vomiting can cause weight changes, dehydration, and malnutrition, which can worsen the overall symptoms of the side effects.

Example: Nana and Lita, my adopted sister had both suffered from nausea and vomiting, but Lita had it worse, it was too bad that she just crawled on the floor crying that "she can't take it anymore, she just wanted to die!"

So, you see, not everybody who gets chemotherapy and radiation has the same symptoms. Some factors of that were the drug they used, the type of cancer and the person itself.

What is the cancer survival rate?

Cancer survival rates or survival statistics tell you the percentage of people who survive a certain type of cancer for a specific amount of time.

These rates are based on research from information gathered on hundreds of thousands of people with specific cancer. An overall survival rate includes people of all ages and health conditions who have been diagnosed with different types cancer, including those diagnosed very early and those very late.

Cancer survival rates often use a five – year survival rate. That doesn't mean cancer can't recur beyond five years. Certain cancers can recur many years after first being found and treated. For some cancers, if it has not recurred by five years after initial diagnosis, the chance of a later recurrence is very small.

However, cancer survival rates can be frustrating. The survival rate for people with your particular cancer might be based on thousands of people. So, while cancer survival rates can give a general idea about most people in your situation, they can't give individual chances for cure or remission. For those reasons, a lot of people ignore cancer survival rate statistics.

It's up to you whether you want to know the survival rates associated with your type and stage of cancer. Because survival rates can't tell you about your situation, you might find the statistics impersonal and not helpful. But some people want to know everything they can about their cancer and their chances of survival.

Knowing more about your cancer can reduce your anxiety as you analyze and choose your options and begin your treatment, but survival statistics can be confusing and frightening.

I don't know about statistics, but five of my loved ones who had been diagnosed with cancer, three didn't make it, two survived. One was in her eleventh year, and the other was in her seven years. Outside my family – my cousin, my nephew's wife, a close friend and a brave young man I was privileged to know. Two died and two survived.

The interesting fact about cancer according to study* Cancer is the second-leading cause of death worldwide. 10 million people die from cancer every year. More than 40%* cancer- related death could be preventable as they are linked to modifiable risk factors such as, smoking, alcohol use, poor diet, physical inactivity and late detection or diagnosis. If we can improve these risk factors maybe we could also cut down unnecessary death.

Chapter 2

You have cancer, what now?

After your healthcare provider told you that you have cancer the first thing that comes to your mind is that you are going to die.

Shock and disbelief are your first reaction to a cancer diagnosis. Often, you feel shock - you may feel numb, as if you aren't feeling any emotion. It may take some time to accept that you have cancer, especially if you don't feel sick; you think you are healthy. This numbness can protect you as you gradually come to terms with the diagnosis. It will take some time for the news to sink in.

Some people may never fully accept the diagnosis. Over time, denial can make it harder to accept the realization that you have cancer and that you are going to die.

Although cancer treatments and outcomes have greatly improved in recent years because of research, modern technologies, and advances in science study, it can still be frightening to hear the word "**cancer**". It's a natural reaction to worry about you having cancer, about the treatment, side effects, test results and the long-term outcome, as well as how your cancer will affect your family, work, responsibilities and finances.

Everybody reacts and copes differently; some people cope better when they learn from their healthcare provider more about the diagnosis and treatment options. The period before a treatment begins can be particularly stressful, but many people feel calmer once treatment is underway.

Anger, guilt and blame

When faced with a cancer diagnosis, it is common to ask, "why me?" You may feel angry with your family or friends, health professionals, the world, God, or even yourself, especially if the cancer is diagnosed late. Cancer often does not cause any symptoms in the early stages, or may be mistaken for other diseases and conditions.

People with cancer often say that their main concern is for the people they love and that they feel guilty about putting them through such a stressful time.

Feeling sad after a cancer diagnosis is common. It is a natural response to loss and disappointment. You may be grieving the way cancer has changed your day-to-day life, your body or your future. If you have continued feelings of sadness, have trouble getting up in the morning, or have lost motivation to do things that previously gave you pleasure, you may be experiencing depression.

Loneliness can lead to depression. Cancer can be isolating, even with many people to support you. You might feel lonely if your family and friends have trouble understanding and coping with your diagnosis, or if you are too sick to work, socialize with others or enjoy your usual activities.

Being told you have cancer can be overwhelming and you may feel that your emotions are spiraling out of control. It may also seem that you are losing control of your life – some people feel helpless or powerless. This can be difficult, especially if you are used to being independent or being the one who takes care of everyone else.

Letting Go, Not Giving Up: Accepting the Reality that you have Cancer

As a person who has not just witnessed someone diagnosed with cancer, but cared for them, found it devastating and overwhelmingly difficult. Perhaps, the hardest part I play is as a witness - watching my loved one wither away, suffering in pain. I feel helpless; I want to do something to alleviate their pain, but there is nothing in God's name that I can do. Sometimes I love them so much that I pray to God to take them away. Stop the suffering; end their life! Unfortunately, that too is out of my hands. So, I have no choice but to bear it and accept it.

To say that learning your loved one had cancer was a shock, is an understatement. You go through different emotions.

You've probably heard about the five stages of grief, which are typically applied to people experiencing the loss of a loved one. We were taught these in school when I was taking a PSW [Personal Support Worker] course. I found these stages therapeutic in learning about and coping with the diagnosis of your loved one to cancer and other debilitating illnesses. Especially when a person is diagnosed with cancer, Alzheimer, or other terminal illnesses, as a young adult, you are most likely experiencing one of the biggest losses of your life.

Stage 1: Denial

My adopted sister had a breast abscess – pus - filled mass of lump on her breast tissue. She had minor surgery done and was advised by her surgeon at Princess Margaret Hospital to have it checked every six months. However, due to hectic schedules - full-time and part-time jobs, she neglected to make an appointment to have it checked. She ignored the symptoms and discomfort she had for years, until one day, she was so sick that I had to beg her to go to the doctor to have it checked. The doctor found a lump and ordered to have it scanned. Less than a week later she received a call from the specialist to come to his office. After she was examined, right away she was ordered to have a biopsy done. After a week, she was asked to report back to his office. It was then that she was finally diagnosed with stage 4 breast cancer with HER2 positive. The type of cancer she had was very invasive and advanced. Her reaction was subdued, and she felt guilty because she almost felt like she'd known it in the back of her mind for a while, and had been denying the reality, because she didn't want this disruption in her life.

Stage 2: Anger

Once the reality of her diagnosis set in, a sense of anger also set in. The hardest part about being diagnosed with cancer is that there is really no one to be angry at but herself for neglecting the symptoms. She carried a lot of anger with her for quite a few weeks, and this anger hasn't quite subsided. It rises to the surface occasionally when she is having a particular bad day. Quite often, this anger stems from the question of "why?" Sometimes she thinks this anger could be relieved if there was a definitive cause of this cancer, so that it could take away the sense of unfairness and regret that she feels.

Stage 3: Bargaining

The bargaining stage is associated with "If only…" statements and imagining how different things might be if only she personally had done something differently. She reflected quite a few times on her lengthy process to diagnosis. More than two years passed from the first breast lump popping up to the beginning of her treatment at which point the tumor had grown to 10.2 cm. She sometimes wonders if things would be different if she had been diagnosed earlier. If her tumor had been smaller at the beginning of her treatment, would she have responded better to her chemo? If she had been diagnosed earlier, would she have less side effects: able to save her breast? Of course, there's no point in lingering on these unanswerable questions that she can't help but think about occasionally.

Stage 4: Sadness and depression

When addressing this stage, it is important to distinguish between sadness and depression. Depression is pervasive and interferes with everyday activities, and recovery can require professional help. Personally, She felt a deep, deep sadness but it never crossed the threshold into depression. It's normal to be sad about a cancer diagnosis. If she starts to count the number of things that she will be missing out of one year and a half treatment, she'll definitely run out of fingers and be broken down in tears by the end of it. For her, the hardest thing to cope with is the thought that she is probably going to die. Going through treatment for cancer doesn't help either, as it's hard to be cheerful while being nauseous, fatigue, and in pain from any number of side effects. But most horrifying is that whenever she looks in the mirror she does not recognize that person in front of her. The most that she can do is look for something positive in everything, and be hopeful that she will survive and beat this cancer. That after the treatment this will all be a memory. Something that has really helped her during this treatment and overcoming the feeling of sadness and loneliness is having me by her side until she finished the treatment and moving forward. By God's grace against all odds, she survived the cancer. It's been twelve long years since she was first diagnosed.

Stage 5: acceptance

Acceptance by no means is defined by letting go of or losing any of the normal emotions that come with a cancer diagnosis. Acceptance, simply means she has made peace with her diagnosis and is ready to put all her energy towards fighting the disease. There came a point where the person with cancer realized that constantly being angry and sad was doing nothing but making her more upset. She realized that in order to beat cancer she was going to need to be strong and accept this as her new [temporary] normal. This doesn't mean she no longer experiences those feelings of sadness, anger, and confusion, but they have become temporary moments rather than persistent moods.

Everyone's journey with cancer is different. Even if you are diagnosed with the same type of cancer as someone you know, your emotions, questions and concerns may be completely different, and it's okay. Having cancer is a deeply personal experience, but that doesn't mean you have to fight it alone. You have to allow and let the people that care and love you to fight with you.

Senya [describe in chapter 3]

thirteen years old diagnosed of Acute Myelogenous Leukemia. Died less than two months after she was diagnosed.

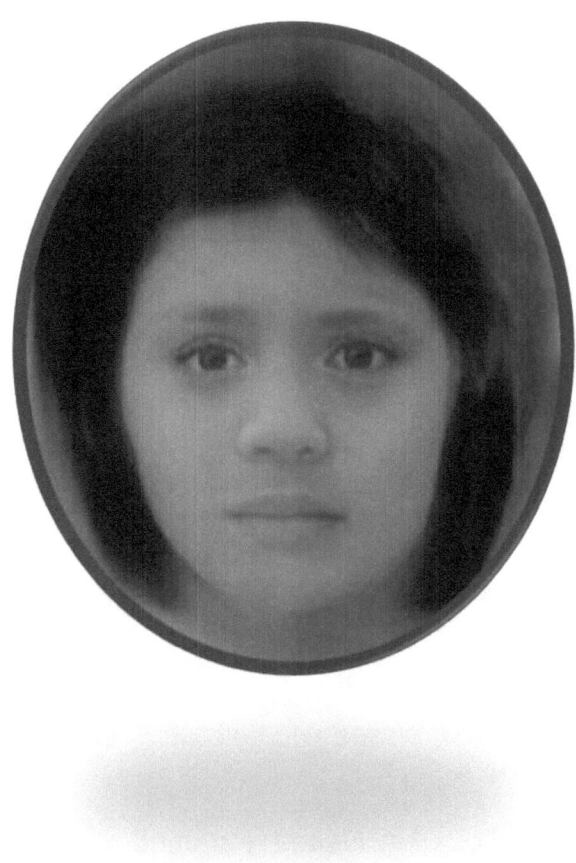

Chapter 3

My first encounter with cancer at a young age

My sister left her family to work as a domestic helper in Hongkong. Her oldest daughter was only nine years old. She was my most favorite niece out of all my nieces, because somehow I felt this connection between us even at the very first time I laid an eye on her when she was born. When my sister put her onto my lap to hold I was delighted. She was beautiful and cute. I was five years older than her, but we were extremely close. I became her confidante – her best friend, and more of a buddy rather than an aunt. She was a very affectionate, loving and very responsible kid. She had assumed the responsibility of caring and rearing for her four younger siblings when her mother left to work abroad. Upon graduation from elementary school, she went to the City to study in a high school, as there was no high school in our place at that time. She would stop over at the house before she went to town, and likewise, on Friday afternoon, after school ended for the weekend. She was always happy to see me. She would embrace me so tightly,

"Auntie, I missed you so much!" she said sadly, almost in tears.

"Are you okay Neng?" I queried.

Something seemed to be wrong, but I couldn't put my finger on it. I had not seen her for a couple of weeks.

36

But she looked like she lost a lot of weight. What was alarming, I noticed some bruising on her hands and legs.

"What's with those bruises?" I asked with concern.

"I don't know auntie, but I had it for some time, not so many in the beginning, but lately it has been showing up. I don't feel well, auntie. I don't know why, but I have had a high temperature for the last two weeks or so, and I have no energy," she said in detail.

Somehow, something hit me. I looked at her more closely, and noted that she looked very pale. I began to panic because as a voracious reader, I had this inkling that something was definitely wrong.

"OMG! Does she have leukemia?" I thought to myself in panic.

I told her to go home and rest, and I will come with her to the City to have her see a doctor. Sunday afternoon she stopped by the house. When I looked at her I was terrified! This time it was very obvious that she was extremely sick.

"I am not going to take you to the doctor. I think you need to go to the hospital to find out what is really wrong with you," I announced.

I went to see her father, and explained that his daughter was very sick and needed to go to the hospital. I packed some clothes for her and other personal needs. We didn't have enough cash, so I told my brother-in-law to take Neneng Senya [that's my niece's name] to Provincial Hospital in Iloilo City [it's a government hospital]. Her great uncle had an office there, as he was an auditor of Health, region six. I figured he could help us in the event that we needed further assistance. Upon arrival at the hospital, we were directed to wait in the Emergency department. There, we were interviewed by a bunch of interns and later by a specialist asking how long she had been sick. I filled them in with as much information that I knew. The doctors and nurses exchanged glances of concern with each other. After a series of tests, I was told that my niece would be given a blood transfusion because her red blood cell count was too low. Actually, a lot more had been explained to me but I was so overwhelmed with all this information coming in that my brain could not process it all at once, not to mention I was scared for what they might find out.

My brother-in-law and I waited patiently. Around ten o'clock in the evening, we were ushered in to sit in one of those cubicles. After half an hour of waiting, two doctors walked in and introduced themselves. One was a hematologist [a specialist in the study of blood, blood-forming organs and blood diseases], and the other was an oncologist [a doctor who has special training in diagnosing and treating cancer].

"We are sorry to inform you of the bad news that your patient has leukemia. She is going to be admitted and we will discuss several options on how we will be going to address her condition," they both uttered, almost in unison.

Shocked to hear the news was an understatement! My worst suspicion had been confirmed. My beloved niece had cancer and she will die.

"How bad is it, doctor? She is too young to have cancer; she is only thirteen years old! Is she going to die?" I asked, crying.

"Your niece has what you call Acute Myelogenous Leukemia. It's a form of leukemia that happens at any age but most common in kids younger than 2 years old and teens. It is a cancer of the blood and the bone marrow. It is the most fatal type of leukemia. Sadly, in your niece's case, the prognosis doesn't look so promising; she is probably in the fourth stage of AML. The only thing that we can do for her is to make her comfortable and reduce the pain. We recommend that she should be in a private room as she is at high risk to get an infection because of her condition if she mixes with other patients," they thoroughly explained.

"You said that she is in the late stage of the disease, and the cure is out of the equation. You talk about making her comfortable. Are you telling us that she is dying? How long then does she have to live?" I asked, afraid to get an answer.

"Depending, but most likely, a patient in her case, 2 to 3 months," they announced without mincing words.

After we left the room I turned to my brother-in-law. I asked him if he understood what was said by the doctors about Neneng Senya's condition. Judging from his reaction I had an inkling that he did not understand the severity of his daughter's illness - that she is dying! I explained everything to him and suggested that we have to let my sister know what's going on. We called my sister in Hongkong and told her everything about her daughter's condition. My sister was heartbroken upon hearing of her daughter's prognosis. There was also guilt that came with it; that if she had not left to work abroad maybe she could have paid more attention to her and none of this would have happened. I tried to console her, but of course it didn't change the fact that her daughter was very sick. Neneng Senya had cancer and was dying!

"Are you coming home Inday Nelly?" I asked.

"Nothing in this world that I would want more than to be with her, Bud's, but if I go home where am I going to get the money to pay for her hospital bills and her other expenses?" she sadly replied.

"I understand your predicament, Inday Nelly, but Neneng Sinya has cancer. She is dying, she could die anytime. I am going to be here for her, but I am not her mother. She needs you!" I said, crying.

I handed the phone to my brother-in-law, and left as I was upset with my sister. I went back to my niece. She looked much better. Her color had come back, more like herself again. Looking at her made me extremely sad. Before I realized it, tears just started to trickle down my cheek. That's when she saw me standing at the foot of her bed.

"Auntie, why were you gone for a long time? I was asking the nurse for you. And why are you crying?" she asked with concern.

"Oh, your father and I were speaking to the doctor about your condition. I am crying because I love you so much and it makes me sad seeing you like this," hugging her tight while speaking.

"I love you too, auntie! What did the doctor say and what is wrong with me?" she asked.

"They are still doing some tests to really determine what is wrong with you. They suggested that you need to be admitted. You will probably be here for a while, Neng." I lied because I was not ready yet to tell her the truth about her condition.

"But, we don't have the money auntie. I don't want to give Nanay another loads to worry about. I feel better now. We can just buy the medicine and I will rest at home," she suggested, not knowing the whole truth about her condition.

My niece, even at a young age, was a very sensible and responsible kid, not to mention, the most affectionate and loving. She became a mother for her younger siblings when her mother left to work for Hong Kong. She was prudent, and frugal; a quality that you rarely see in teenagers her age. She would save her allowance that her father gave her for the week, so that she could have money to buy a present for her younger siblings when she came home on weekends. She is so beautiful inside and out. I am not saying this because she is my niece, but she is really beautiful. She is tall, morena [dark], long, natural luster, long hair, big black bright eyes, long lashes, nice brows, symmetric nose, full perky cheeks and a well-defined jawline. Even the doctors and nurses at the emergency noticed it – nakakapanghinayang… [it's sad, regrettable], they all commented.

My niece was admitted to the hospital into a semi private room [two patients in one room]. Her father went home as he needed to earn a living and take care of the younger children. I had discussed with him about telling Neneng Senya the truth about her condition. He was okay with it; he gave me the task of telling it to her.

The first three weeks that we were there at the hospital, she was stable; the pain was manageable by painkillers and she got blood transfusions once a week, but then things started to get worse. She started to have nose bleeds and had high temperatures very often. She was constantly in pain. Watching her groaning, crying, and calling my name to help her, I felt like I was in a torture chamber; it is excruciating to watch your loved one suffer, you want to help but there is nothing that you can do. You are helpless! Making it more difficult was the problem that her blood type was one of the rare types, AB+. The blood bank had run out of blood because that's the only place we could go to get blood and she was getting a blood transfusion twice a week. We had all our immediate family, close relatives and people we knew tested, but none had her blood type match, not even her father. We even went to a prison facility to ask the prisoners if they wanted to be tested and willing to donate their blood for some amount. We were lucky to have found two. But that's only good for a week. I had my blood type tested, and to my delight I had the same blood type as her – type AB+.

"No wonder we have a special bond, because we have the same blood type," I thought to myself.

But things were not that simple. I could not give my blood to her without my parents' permission as I was still a minor. I could not leave my niece alone in the hospital to go home and get my parents' consent, so, I had no choice but to forge my parents' signatures. After I presented my parents' consent, the nurse checked my vital signs and explained to me the procedure. I was told that it was going to be an **"indirect transfusion"**, meaning I would be giving my blood from my vein then stored in a blood bag which would then be transfused into my niece immediately. I lay beside her, amazed how my blood was being transported from my vein to her vein. After she received my blood, she was okay, maybe for a day. Then she started bleeding again, this time not just from her nose, but also the blood coming from her ear and sometimes when she peed and pooped. I could see that she was terrified, and suspected there was more to the story about her illness than what we were telling her.

"Auntie, please tell me the truth, what is wrong with me?" she asked.

Before I could answer her, I took a long deep breath to prepare myself, or rather find some courage and strength to tell her the truth.

"Neng, you have leukemia. That's the reason that you have these bruises, high temperatures and bleeding. Also, the reason that you are getting a blood transfusion is because your blood cells are not giving you healthy blood cells because you have cancer of the blood, or leukemia," I explained in tears.

"Am I going to die, auntie?" she asked, crying.

"According to the doctor, your prognosis doesn't look good. Your cancer is in the last stage of the disease," I said, hugging her tight, afraid to let her go.

"Auntie, don't cry! I am going to get better. I don't want to die yet. Please help me auntie...!" she asked, holding me tight.

"Of course, Neng. You know that I would do anything for you because you are my niece and I love you so much," reassuring her.

In spite of knowing the truth about her condition, it didn't deter her. Instead, she was even more determined to live. She strived so hard to beat the cancer, she forced herself to eat even when she was throwing up or in excruciating pain. She kept a positive attitude to help her through it, but in the end I could see that we were losing the battle. It was heart wrenching for me to watch her slowly wither away. I believe cancer is harder on the loved ones than it is on those who have cancer.

"Auntie, I want to fight but I am so tired now. I had no more energy left in me. I am tired of the needles, of the pain. I want to be a free auntie. I want to rest now," she uttered in a melancholic voice.

"Neng, I wish that I could take that load off your shoulder and carry it for you but I can't. I wish too, that you would win this battle and you will once again be a healthy young girl, but I have no power. My only wish at this moment for you is not to suffer anymore. I love you so much, but if it means staying makes you endure more suffering, then I don't want that. So, even if it breaks my heart, it is okay for you to go if you are tired already," telling her in tears.

"Auntie, I want to see nanay [mother]before I die," she uttered in anguish.

"I will try my very best Neng, I will call your mother and tell her your dying wishes," I said. I was overwhelmed with sadness.

44

We sat in bed, holding each other tight and crying, I don't know how long. Both of us were silent. Honestly, what is there to say? Nothing, really! Looking at her made me so mad. She was only thirteen years old for Pete's sake! She is a good kid; responsible, acquiescent and dutiful. She was smart, a good student. She dreamt to be a flight stewardess, and travel across the globe. Unfortunately, her hopes and dreams for the future got snatched away from her too early by cancer. She was robbed too early of the life she could have had. Sometimes it is easier for me to feel bitter, sad and angry, than it was to accept the reality that my sweet niece was dying; soon she would be leaving me.

I waited for the doctor's rounds to hear what they had to say. My niece's oncologist was very nice and very empathetic towards her; he always spent time with her, asking her how she feels.

"*Good morning! How's my favorite patient?*" he greeted her with a big smile.

"*I have accepted my fate, doctor. That said, I don't want to have a blood transfusion anymore,*" she said with conviction, looking her doctor in the eyes with a forceful smile.

He gave my niece a gentle squeeze on her shoulder and told me to follow him as he wanted to discuss things without my niece hearing. He was forthright, yet very empathetic. He told me that my niece did not have that much time; maybe a week, a couple of weeks. All the lab results and vital signs don't look good at all. He gave me instructions on how to care for her;

I called my sister, and relayed what was her daughter's dying wish. I explained to her that Neneng Senya doesn't have that much time left. So, if she decides to come home she should do it right away, as time is of the essence. She promised me that she will try her best; she is going to talk to her employer, and she will let me know. My heart goes out for my sister, it must have been agonizing for her to know that her beloved daughter was in the final stages of a difficult and painful death.

The next day, my brother-in-law came by and told us that my sister was coming home to see her daughter for a week- as that's the only time her employer allowed her to have. It's really short, but it is better than nothing. The most important thing is that she will see her daughter. Neneng Senya was so happy to know that her mother was coming home.

"Auntie, can you buy me Dinuguan [a Filipino dish made of blood, meat and some organs]? she asked affectionately.

"Yes of course, anything for you!" I said almost in shock because she had not eaten solid food for a week - just soup and fruits.

My niece was the most positive person I knew; she never complained nor asked "why" she got cancer? She accepted her fate. She was beyond her years, she bore the pain, the needles, fought with every fiber of her being, every ounce of her body to beat this cancer, but in the end she knew that she was losing the battle, and she accepted that her life was nearly over. It was heart wrenching for me to watch my beautiful niece turn into almost a skeleton - bones covered with skin. It was gut-wrenching!!!

My sister and my brother-in-law came around eight o'clock in the evening straight from the airport. My sister was inconsolable to see her daughter in that state. She held her so tight; almost breaking her fragile bones.

"Nay [mother], don't cry anymore. We have to accept that this is my fate. I love you and tatay [father], and also my siblings. I don't want you to be sad when I am gone because if you do I will be sad too where I am going," she said so affectionately.

I had to leave the room because it was heartbreaking to watch the two of them, even the nurses and our roommate [bed next to us] were also in tears.

After my sister and my brother-in-law left, my niece was quiet. I knew her very well more than anyone else. I knew something was bothering her.

"Are you okay Neng, what's with the sad face? I thought you would be happy to see your mother" I asked.

"Nothing, auntie. I just thought that mother would stay with me tonight because I missed her so much. But I understand that she has to see my brothers and sisters too." She said with pain visible in her face.

I didn't say anything or offer an opinion. But I totally understood how she felt. I voiced my opinion when I was alone with my sister. I told her without mincing words or sugarcoating how I thought. After all, the reason for her coming home was to spend time with her dying daughter. But then again, I don't know how she was feeling inside. I can't just imagine…must be excruciating!

A day before my sister was due to go back to Hongkong, she came to the hospital with a witch doctor, a relative of my brother-in-law. She claimed that my niece was cursed by goblins because her father destroyed their house and killed the son of the goblin. To get back at my brother-in-law he cursed my niece and said she will die unless she gets out of the hospital and does the ritual to appease the goblins. I was livid watching her perform her ritual on my niece. I confronted my sister over it.

"Inday Nelly, I understand where you're coming from because I love Neneng Sinya too, and I will do anything if there is a chance that she will live. But Neneng Senya has cancer, and she is dying. If she is discharged in this hospital she will not survive a day. She doesn't have that much time to live, why don't we just let her be. We owe it to her to die in comfort and peacefully," pleading with her.

"Bud's I am sorry, but I want to explore other avenues. She is in this hospital for almost two months, instead of getting better she has gotten worse. I will not accept that my daughter is going to die. She is too young to die! So why don't we try other alternatives. How about if Sidra [name of the witch doctor] is right that Neneng Senya was indeed cursed? At this point in time, we have nothing to lose, but to gain," she said firmly, her mind made up.

Against my will, I had no choice but to comply. I was in no position to criticize my sister. I just couldn't imagine the anguish that my sister must be going through inside. Once again she left for Hong Kong, as her employer only gave her one week. The next day I talked to her oncologist that the family wanted to have her discharged. And Neneng Sinya wanted to go home to see her siblings before she died, [I didn't tell the doctor about the witchcraft]. He was very understanding; he gave me advice on what to do and gave me prescriptions for morphine and how to administer it if she had pain. Before we left Neneng Senya's oncologist and the nurses said their goodbyes to her and they all wished her good luck!

On the way home in the car, the witch doctor was with us – chanting, doing her ritual with her. In the meantime, my niece was groaning in pain, bleeding [nose and ear], and the bumpy road was making it worse; lots of sinkholes, besides from the fact that it was a long journey home; about twenty-seven kilometers from the city proper to our house in the countryside. She was taken straight to the house of their leader in Batuyanan [Pulahan cult]. There, they carried her inside, chanting, [all kinds of nonsense]. If it weren't enough, she let her drink the blood of the [black] pig that they just slaughtered, which according to her was the offering asked by the goblins to appease them. I was furious and livid when I saw that she was whipping my niece with a sprig and started shaking her. I went berserk! I went off the deep end.

"Will you stop doing that to my niece! Can't you see you are killing her? She is dying!" I blurted, enraged!

"Buday, you are interfering with my job. If you want to stay, be quiet, but if you can't control yourself, leave! Because I am trying to save Neneng Senya's life," she retorted.

To avoid the squabbles and not have my niece caught in the middle, I decided to leave to take a breathing space; otherwise, I might do something that I might regret. Looking at her I didn't know if I would see her alive when I got back. I planted a kiss on her forehead and whispered in her ears.

"Neng, I love you so much! I am sorry that I have to leave you, but I have to, before I will do something that I might regret," telling her in tears.

"Auntie, please don't leave me...I love you auntie. Thank you for everything!" she said, tears streaming off her face.

I ran from there, as fast as I could. It tore my heart apart, because this should not have happened. She should have been in the hospital, in bed, comfortable in her last remaining hours of her life. Instead, she was paraded for a long journey for some gibberish ritual!

I went to my aunt's house to calm down and relax before I went back to my niece. But I was anxious and restless. I kept hearing her voice calling my name, so, after half an hour I went back, but I was heartbroken to find her dead. Her lifeless body lay on the floor. Seeing her condition, I lost it! I chased the "witch", told her to stay out of my sight because if I see her again I will have her head cut off and offer it to the goblins myself.

I held my niece's lifeless body for a while. No one could remove me from her. I don't know if I should be happy that finally her suffering has ended. However, knowing that I will never see that sweet smile, that calming voice again, her lovely face brought a flurry of pain and extreme sadness in my heart.

I think the magnitude of this can be hard to recognize when looking at it from the outside in, and I think those who experience the losses are often surprised by how hard "acceptance" is when you care deeply about someone. It can be difficult to let go and accept that the person you love and care so much is no longer around.

Nana [describe in chapter 4]

Diagnosed of Ovarian Cancer, stage 4. Lived for three years after been told to have only 2 – 4 months to live before she finally succumbed to her death.

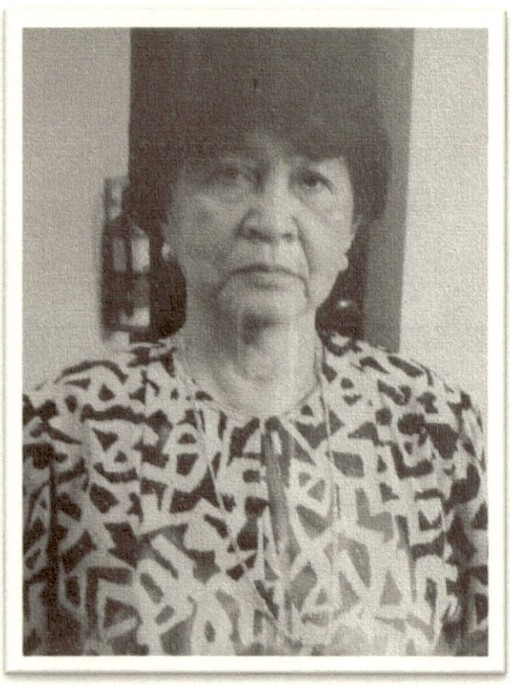

Chapter 4

Without warning

When I lost my mother, at the age of fifty-seven, I was devastated. This was this big hole in my heart that went with her. It took me a long time to recover from it, mostly the guilt of not being there for her and regrets for not being able to make up for what I put her through during my childhood and teen years.

But when Nana Carling came to Canada, she filled the void of my longing for my mother. She took care of me like her own. She was my alarm clock, she prepared my lunch box, woke up early in the morning to prepare my breakfast before I went to work and she did my laundry for me. She would wait for me when I came home around midnight, with my favorite drink - tea with lemon and honey waiting on the table for me. She would tiptoe in the wee hours of the night to check if I had a blanket on me. In other words, she was a mother whom I longed for – she was a very special person in my life.

One summer, she went home to the Philippines for a month and half. When I picked her up at the airport, I noticed that she lost a lot of weight and somehow her eyes seemed dull and lifeless. There is a saying that, "our eyes are the mirror of one's soul", we can lie about feeling okay or happy but our eyes will certainly reveal the truth. And also, the phrase "our eyes are the window to the soul" is the idea that you can understand a person's emotions and sometimes thoughts by just merely looking into his or her eyes.

"Nana, are you feeling okay?" I asked her with concern.

"I am okay, except that my stomach seemed heavy and bloated all the time" she replied.

"I am going to make an appointment for you to see Dr. L, [we have the same GP] so that he can give you something for indigestion" I remarked!

She had just come back to Canada from the Philippines on the weekend. The following Thursday at dawn, she went to the washroom to peed, she was frightened when she looked at the toilet - there was a lot of fresh blood that came with her pee. She called us to show what's in there; lots of fresh blood alright! I called our GP right away, pleading for an appointment for her. I described what transpired with Nana. Two hours later, his secretary whom I befriended over the years of going there; I had been a patient of this doctor for twenty years. He is the kindest and most empathetic doctor I had ever known. He is attentive, and always listens to your opinion and respects it.

"Loretta, just bring her over around 12:30, once Dr. L is done with all his patients he will see your aunt," she explained.

"Thank you so much, Sara. I am extremely grateful for accommodating us," I said relieved.

We arrived at the doctor's clinic earlier than we were told to come. Even Sara expressed concern upon seeing her; she commented that Nana lost a lot of weight. An hour later, Dr. L called us into one of those cubicles to examine Nana; he concentrated on her lower abdomen, below the belly button, and pelvis. I can see that he was concerned because every time he pressed those areas Nana grimaced in pain. After he examined her, he sent Nana to have an ultrasound. And told me that he had asked for the result ASAP and asked me to call the office on the following Monday.

In the meantime, over the weekend Nana's stomach just got bigger; she looked like six months pregnant. She was very uncomfortable, could not eat and experienced shortness of breath and was also in pain the whole weekend.

First thing Monday morning, I called Dr. L's clinic and left a message to call me as soon as they had the result of the ultrasound as I was very anxious because Nana's condition had gotten worse. Around 10:25 in the morning, I received a call from Dr. L, himself requesting me to come to his office to discuss the result of the ultrasound. I dropped everything and went over to his clinic. Sarah asked me to sit down and wait for the doctor to call me. Half an hour later, I was ushered into his office.

"Loretta, the result of the ultrasound showed that there was fluid accumulation there, but the radiologist cannot determine where it's coming from. She recommended that your aunt have a CT scan to confirm her suspicion," he explained

"Cancer? The passing of blood, her stomach got bigger in just two days, her sudden loss of weight and her general physical appearance, I am afraid she might have cancer." I expressed concern.

"I will send her for a CT scan to really determine where those fluids are coming from. I will ask Sara to fax the requisition but if you don't hear from them after

two days, give them a call to follow up," he said with empathy.

"Thank you so much, doctor. Please help us to speed up the CT scan appointment and for my aunt to get help," I pleaded.

"I will try my best, Loretta. I am sorry; hopefully, if it's turned out to be cancer let's hope that it's still curable. If her condition gets worse, take her to the emergency," he furthered advice.

After I thanked doctor L, I left his office perturbed and sad, thinking about Nana. She was still young; only sixty-seven. I uttered a simple prayer for her asking God to spare her and give her strength to face whatever is ahead. After two days I didn't hear from the CT scan, so I gave them a call to follow-up Nana's appointment, but was disappointed to find out that her appointment wouldn't be for another month. I explained that she didn't have that luxury to wait because of her condition which is deteriorating by the day and she may not be alive to get to that appointment. The gravity of her illness means that time was of the essence; a CT scan plays a crucial role in helping determine the correct diagnosis. An accurate diagnosis is critical to prevent wasting precious time on the wrong course of treatment.

"I am sorry to hear about your aunt, but we have a long backlog. The only thing that I can do is to put her on the cancellation list." She said sound sympathetic.

I was appreciative of the CT scan receptionist's effort to help; putting Nana on the "cancellation" list. But what if no one canceled, which means she had no choice but to wait for her appointment which is another month.

After pondering over it, I called doctor L again to ask for his help on what to do. Even he thought that a month was way too long to wait. He suggested taking Nana to the emergency department at Sunnybrook Hospital. Thinking about it, I thought that was a fantastic idea! I asked one of her daughters to come with me just in case I may need some back-up as I have to go to work in the afternoon. We arrived at the emergency department at 4:30 in the morning, enough time for me to assist Nana and talk to the doctors and answer questions they may have before I went to my work. After a long hour of waiting, she was finally seen by the doctor at the emergency department at 9:15 am. I told them everything from the beginning: the passing of fresh blood in her pee, her stomach getting bigger, the sudden drop of weight and not being able to eat because she feels uncomfortable and in a lot of pain. I even exaggerated a bit. Nana underwent a series of tests: Complete Blood Test [CBC], Basic Metabolic Panel, Blood Enzymes and Bleeding Parameters; they had taken five vials of blood in which every tube of blood has a specific purpose. She had a CT scan done, and finally the oncologist performed Paracentesis. He explained to me that the procedure is to drain the excess fluid from her peritoneal cavity. He inserted a small tube into the abdomen and drained off the fluid to reduce the swelling and also to make her feel comfortable. He drained 3 liters of fluid from Nana's abdomen. Looking at those yucky looking fluids that were coming out from her, I felt the worse was coming. I have an inquisitive mind by nature and always ask questions, especially things I don't understand. I asked the doctors to please explain to me what exactly was going on. I had been told that they will send the ascitic fluid taken from her abdomen to the lab for testing. So, we would find out in a few hours the result of those tests: blood work, CT scan, and the ascites fluid. The doctor was very forthright with me; things didn't look good. I left my work number, to call me as soon as they had the results, or anything else they needed to ask me. When Nana heard that I was leaving for work she appeared anxious. Somehow, she feels secure when I am there, not that she doesn't trust her daughters to take care of her, just that she knows how persistent I can become and I never shy away from asking questions if there are things I don't understand. Her daughters were very good children; they all loved her, but they were a quiet type – laid back.

"Nana, don't worry I am going to work but I will keep in touch with the doctor. I left them my number and the minute they have the results of your CT scan and lab results they will call me. I will come here after work." Trying to reassure her anxious mind.

I went to work distracted, but I tried to focus on the work at hand. I believe that my problem at home, stays at home. And my problem at work, stays at work. My residents should not be affected by my personal problems for they deserve the best care that I can give them. I had just finished putting my residents to bed when my charge nurse called me and said that I had a phone call. It was the doctor at Sunnybrook - head of Geriatric Palliative Care Department. He wanted to see me to discuss Nana's prognosis. According to him, it was confirmed it is cancer- cancer of the ovary. I was speechless there for a second or two. Just cried! I told him that I would not be finished until eleven in the night. He told me that he will wait for me. He gave me direction on how to get to his office at Sunnybrook. My peers and charge nurse were so empathetic of my situation that they allowed me to go home earlier.

When I got to the doctor's office, he asked me to sit down. I was told that Nana is in the last stage of Ovarian cancer. It had already metastasized; the disease had spread out to other organs and tissues. That explained why there was lots of fluid accumulating in her abdomen. According to him surgery was out of the question as it had already spread out. Chemo, he didn't think that it would help her; it would just prolong her suffering. The best thing for her was to be comfortable and die with dignity. He would facilitate a Palliative care team to come to the house – doctor, nurse, social worker and PSW to help assist with her ADL [activity of daily living]. He would send a referral to CCAC [Community Care Access Center], and he would also send the report to my family doctor to contact the CCAC supervisor in charge of Nana's case. I was overwhelmed with all this information coming rapidly that I sat, flustered and dejected.

"Doctor, please don't tell me that you are giving up on her?" I asked, upset.

"This is not the question of giving up, but it's about fact. We are only doctors, not miracle workers." He replied.

"So, how long does she have then?" I asked sadly.

"Based on her prognosis, probably 2 to 4 months," he answered unequivocally.

After I thanked him, walking in that dark corridor all the way to Nana's room seemed eternal. As I opened the door, she smiled when she saw me, her three daughters were by her sides [Lita, Janet and Libeth].

"Hello Nana! How are you feeling?" I asked.

"Much, much better. My stomach is much lighter and it doesn't hurt anymore when I eat; unlike before." She answered smiling.

"Nana, would you mind if we [Lita and Janet], leave you for a bit as we have some papers to sign at the doctor's office. Libeth [another daughter who is mentally challenged] will stay with you," I said, lying.

She nodded at me with approval. Lita, Janet and I went outside the room and I told them everything that the doctor told me about Nana's prognosis. They both cried uncontrollably upon hearing. They both suggested not telling her, but I was against it, as Nana deserves to know the truth; after all it is her life. After contemplating about it, they both agreed with me that Nana deserves to know the truth. It was decided that I am the one to tell her. We got back into Nana's room.

"How am I going to tell this bitter truth about her condition, not alone to tell her that the doctor has given her only 2-4 months to live? But I have no choice; she has to know," I thought to myself.

After I told her everything that there is to know, she was silent, not a word that came out of her mouth.

"Nana, are you okay? What am I saying of course you're not okay!" Lita, Janet and me holding her hands.

"So, Am I going to die?" she asked dejectedly.

"Nana, listen to me, doctors are not God! We promised you this that we will not give up on you. We

will explore every avenue; leave no stone unturned and we will do humanly possible to get you some help. However, we don't want to give you false hope, we will do everything but then again God has the last say about our fate, so we have to prepare ourselves for whatever His will for us. Nana, you pray and surrender everything to Him; who is the author of life and death," comforting and encouraging her not to lose hope.

"I trust you Lori. I know you will do everything to help me. Please guide Lita and Janet as they are not stronger like you are," she uttered with tears in her eyes.

Nana was discharged from Sunnybrook. The next few days I was busy arranging things for her to be comfortable at home. Dr. L called me to express empathy and told me that he had sent the request of palliative care at home to CCAC, and I would be hearing from the supervisor in charge of her case. Within a span of forty-eight hours, everything had been arranged: the Case manager in charge of her case, have nurses comes every day to check on her, PSW [Personal Support Worker], to help her with bathing and prepare her meal, social worker to address her emotion, Palliative doctor to come to the house if the fluid starts to accumulate in her abdomen, and scheduled a hospital bed to be delivered in the house for Nana. In other words, everything has been in place. Thank God for Canada! Sometimes, we take for granted what we have in Canada. What we do not realize is how lucky we are to be living in this beautiful country. Yes, our healthcare system is not perfect, nevertheless, Canadians can count on their government to take care of them in time of their needs. Canadians do likewise share important values such as pride, a belief in equality and diversity, and respect for all individuals. It is these values that make Canada known as a friendly, peace loving, and secure place in which to live.

My shift at work starts at 3 o'clock and finishes at 11 in the night, but I worked part-time in the morning for 5 hours doing private clients. Since Nana came home from the hospital, she has been tapped [drained]; to take the fluid off her abdomen about 3x. After I finished my part-time job, I went home to check on her. Found her in the dark; all the blinds were closed, and refused to eat or do anything. She was crying. She thought that we don't care about her because we still go to work while she is alone with Libeth.

"Nana, we need to work because we have bills to pay and we need money to put food on the tables. What do you want us to do, sit in the dark with you and stop living? Is that it? I said opening all the blinds.

"I am sorry Lori, but of all people, why me? I am afraid to die. I don't want to die yet! Please help me Lori," pleading with me in tears.

"Nana, I am sorry to have raised my voice on you. But I need you to be strong, to fight with me. I cannot do this alone on my own. Do you hear me?" challenging her.

"I promised Lori! I will try to be strong," she said in tears.

I gave her a shower, and food to eat- she didn't eat that much. Then I called Dr. L to get a second opinion. If it turns out that the diagnosis was the same, then at least I would have this peace of mind that I can explore other avenues. He was very understanding about my desire for a second opinion. He gave me the name of the doctor from Princess Margaret [a well-known cancer hospital in Canada] to call. I did not waste any time at all; I called the doctor right away. It was a voice recorder, what's new? "In this day and age" we hardly speak to humans when we call. I left a message and my contact number begging for this doctor to call me. Surprisingly, after an hour or so, the secretary had called me to book an appointment. When I told her that we live in Markham, she told me that I don't have to come to Princess Margaret as this doctor had an office in Markham Stouffville hospital, I was pleased because it's just a 3 minutes' drive from home. She booked an appointment for Nana in less than two weeks, but upon learning the doctor schedules at Markham Stouffville I devised a plan; hopeful that it may work to accelerate her seeing this doctor. At this critical juncture of Nana's illness, I am willing to try everything. Anyway, I have nothing to lose, the worst that could happen is we go home empty handed'.

"Nana, we are going fishing to catch a 'fat fish' in the hospital." I said smiling.

"What? You don't make sense Lori." She exclaimed!

After I explained everything to her, that we are going to the emergency at Markham Stouffville, hoping to catch this doctor that probably would be the answer to our prayers - second opinion and hope for her. She was ecstatic upon hearing it; she got ready in no time. We arrived at the emergency around five am. She was not seen by the doctor until nine am. She was examined by an internist, asked me what was wrong with her.

Told him everything that she has Ovarian cancer, discharged by Sunnybrook hospital and transferred her care to the palliative care team. He was a bit rude, asked me why then, didn't I call her palliative doctor instead of taking her to the emergency room. I replied because she was extremely sick; throwing up, and groaning for pain the whole night. She was not able to eat nor drink the whole day and night. He left the room without saying anything. We waited, and waited for hours, until finally, the door opened and a man, maybe in mid sixty with a "bowtie" walked in.

"Hello, my name is Doctor S. I am a Pathologist and Oncologist in this hospital. I gathered that your mother was discharged from Sunnybrook. First of all, would you sign the paper requesting for them to release all her medical records so that I can review it?" He said smiling.

"Absolutely doctor!" I uttered in excitement.

Nana signs the document requesting Sunnybrook to release all her medical records. He left after taking the paper from Nana, but promised to be back in an hour or so after he reviewed her medical record. After an hour and a half, he appeared at the door.

"I have finished reviewing all her lab tests and prognosis, and there is no doubt that she had Ovarian cancer. I am going to do a biopsy to confirm the grade and stages of the cancer. Once that is confirmed I will design the right treatment for her - what kind of chemo-drug I will use to treat your mother. In the meantime, I will prescribe her the pills to slow down the growth of cancer, while she is waiting for her chemotherapy. If all her blood tests and liver function tests are normal, then I will prepare her for chemo treatment right away. She

64

needs to have a complete blood work. And I need you and your mother to attend a class about chemotherapy so that you have a well-informed understanding about the chemo: the drugs, the treatment and the side effects. Do you have any questions?" he asked, looking at Nana.

"Not at the moment doctor. Although I am astounded by what I am hearing from you, it's the opposite of what the doctor from Sunnybrook had told us – Nana has no more hope; he gave her 2-4 months to live. Whereas, you on the other hand are giving her a ray of hope. Thank you so much doctor, you are an answer to our prayers." I was overwhelmed with joy.

"I am a doctor; my job is to help people in any way I can. It's not my job to say how long my patient will live, that's for God to determine, not mine. By that said, the treatment that I am giving your mother will not guarantee a positive result, I will do my best to help her but your mother needs to pray for I am merely an instrument by God," he honestly uttered.

Nana was extremely overjoyed and hopeful that maybe she gets another chance of life. After she finished with all the tests needed we stopped by at the pharmacy to get her prescription. After a couple of days, I received a call from the doctor's secretary, asking me to come the following day to attend the "Chemotherapy patient education". I took a days' off from work and Nana was very excited to go-woke up very early in the morning.

The nurses at the chemo treatment and the team of oncology nurses were the one giving the education. It was very informative - told us about chemotherapy, whom to call for healthcare support; management and prevention of side effects; importance of and tools for adherence and safety issues. After we finished we were handed a chemotherapy patient education booklet to read. We were told that Nana's treatment will start in a week. She will receive 7 cycles of treatment; she will get a continuous infusion for 7 days, then 3 weeks rest is one cycle. She will be using the chemo drugs Paclitaxel [Taxol] and the platinum- based drug Carboplatin.

After two weeks of chemotherapy, Nana has started to get a severe side effect: sore on her mouth, nausea; throwing up, and one day I was giving her a shower when a chunk of her hair fell off. But it is no surprise, for we've been told that these might have happened as the effects of the chemotherapy. I shaved off her hair and Lita bought her a wig to wear. I kept encouraging Nana to keep a positive attitude; it is the only way to help her through it. Mind you, she was tough and very strong, but sometimes no matter how strong you were the treatment sapped your strength; you feel completely wiped out.

Treatment it's like a baby step…will you walk, can you run, and how long will it last? The fear, the wondering, just moving through the motions of treatment is the most difficult journey of your life.

Finally, Nana's had completed her seven cycles of chemotherapy. The nurses rang the bells and congratulated her for her great accomplishment. It meant the end of a tough chapter of chemotherapy was over. Nana expressed gratitude to everyone who were there: nurses, volunteers and doctors

The tradition started in 1996 at MD Anderson, A rear Admiral in the U. S. Navy, Irve Le Moyne, was undergoing radiation therapy for head and neck cancer, and he told his doctor that he planned to follow a Navy tradition of ringing a bell to signify "when the job is done." He brought a brass bell to his treatment, and rang it several times. And left it as a donation. Later, it was mounted on a wall plaque with the inscription:

Ringing out

Ring this bell

Three times well

It's toll to clearly say, My treatments done

This course is run

And I am on my way!

-Irve Le Moyne

After the treatment, doctor S saw Nana. According to him, Nana was responding to chemotherapy. All tests and blood work were normal. The last thing to confirm if she is truly cancer free is the CT scan. He scheduled Nana to have a PET/CT scan after 12 weeks. Then he will see her again to discuss the result. In the meantime, he advised Nana to try to return to normalcy. *"Sometimes the treatment can be as rough as the disease."* But the bottom line, she was able to overcome it. Before cancer, Nana was a very active, full of life woman. She walked every day with her best friend, Manang Alma; who lived a few houses from us. She was also a member of a Filipino retired men and women who traveled by "tour bus" going to places, excursions and Casinos. We encouraged her to try and get back to her old life since she was feeling a lot better. Her stomach just went down, she hasn't had an ascites tap for more than two months. Her appetite and strength were slowly coming back. After two months and a half, she had her PET/CT scan. After a week we went to see doctor S, and we were euphoric: extremely happy and excited upon hearing that Nana was "cancer free". In excitement I gave doctor S a hug. I was over the moon! For someone that has been told to just have 2-4 months to live, it is a miracle indeed! Her Children were crying when I told them the good news.

After three years of life after cancer, Nana can't believe she could get back to feeling 100% normal again after what she had been through. She didn't think it was possible, even doctor L cannot believe it, but she did!

Summer of 2010, they just got back from a trip from Midland church with her group. When she arrived home, she complained of pain in her abdomen. She further added that she was feeling nauseous and bloated. I was alarmed because when I looked at her closely, I was terrified! I saw that same look on her eyes when I picked her up at the airport prior to her being diagnosed with cancer.

I did not waste any time. right away I left a message for doctor S for an appointment to see Nana, describing what was happening with her. We got an appointment the following week. He examined her and requested for her to have a CT scan the next day. After two days, I received a call from her secretary to come to the office to discuss the CT scan result.

"I am terribly sorry to tell you that your mother's cancer has come back!" he uttered without doubt.

Upon hearing it, I was heartbroken. My thought was with Nana, how the heck would I break this news to her- that her cancer had come back? I composed myself and asked him.

"What now doctor?" I asked feeling jittery

"We will try to put her back on chemotherapy. Let's hope to God that it will work like the first time. I will use the same drugs Paclitaxel [Taxol], and a combination of Carboplatin. We will start her with four cycles, see how she will respond," he said.

When I got home, I gathered her daughters [three of them here in Toronto], and one in California. I told them exactly what doctor S had said. Unfortunately, Nana's cancer came back! We went to her room and broke the news. She was devastated, she was speechless for a while. A cancer recurrence can bring back many of the same emotions you felt when you were first diagnosed with cancer.

"Nana, we are sorry that you have to go through with this again. If you would like to talk about it, we are all here for you. You're not alone in this journey. We will be with you every step of the way, like before," Trying to comfort her.

She did not say anything, she just cried. But what is there really to say? Nothing!

She was on her second cycle of chemo treatment when doctor S had to stop because she was not responding to treatment. Her abdomen started to blow up again like she was seven months pregnant. She lost a lot of weight, as she couldn't eat well. We were back and forth in the hospital. Doctor S called me to say that he is going to try another chemo drug called Docetaxel again with the combination of platinum agent-

Carboplatin. She had just finished first cycle when a long list of side effects appeared: the most common side effects are the dropping of red and white blood cells, difficulty breathing, water retention, infection, nausea and vomiting, fever and chill and the list goes on… in other word, Nana was a mess. The unfortunate thing about chemo is it kills more than it helps. Literally it becomes a race if it is going to kill you first, or the cancer.

On October 10, 2010, Nana succumbed to her death after a long journey of fighting the disease. She fought it valiantly-with great courage and determination. She died peacefully surrounded by her loved one with a clear mind.

Finally, she rested from constant poking of needles, endless blood tests, ultrasound, and CT scan. She is at peace now, in a better place; no pain and suffering with His creator.

We grieved for her death of course. For myself I felt like Déjà vu; losing a mother again. Grief is a person's spiritual, emotional, intellectual and physical reaction to loss. What helps me in coping with Nana's death is my faith in God; knowing that I am never alone. His loving care always lifts me up, countering the depressing effects of my loss. The warmth of His love continually radiates my spirit and it helps to bring my consciousness out of the cold and dark of loss into His presence again. It gives me the strength and courage to move on.

I had peace because wherever Nana was, she knew that we did try our best to get her all the help she needed. She may be dead but her lasting memory will forever stay in our heart.

Lita [describe in chapter 5]

Diagnosed of Invasive breast cancer HER2 positive, stage 3. After a long and difficult journeyed of treatments and coping with side effects, she is an "alivers" of cancer. It's been 12 years since she was diagnosed. She is determined, not let cancer define her rather she enjoys every moment of her life.

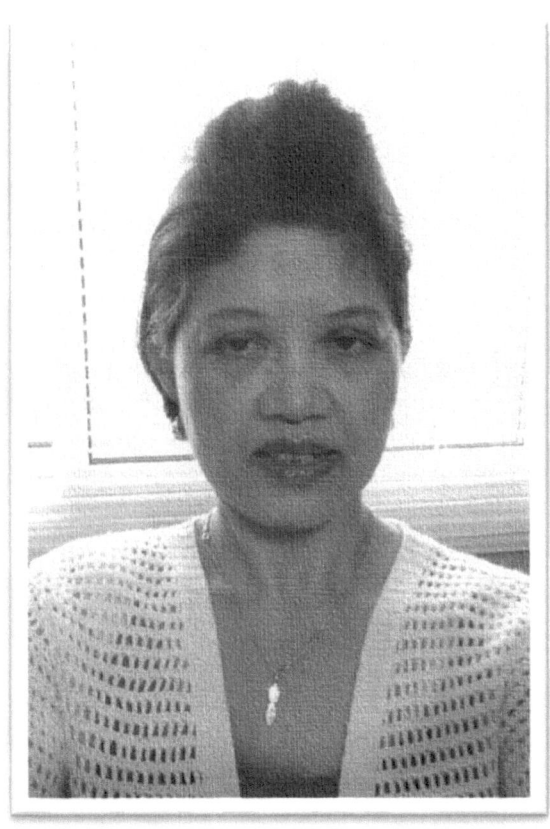

Chapter 5

A long journey to recovery

Lita and I had known each other way back since when we were in Hong Kong. I met her when I was at the very lowest point of my life. She was there for me, lifted me up and brought me back from the abyss I was in and most of all she returned me back to God. She was there for me in every adversity I faced; holding my hands, encouraged me to keep going and never gave up. She stood up for me and defended me to everyone who would hurt me. She is honest, always speaks from the heart; tells me what I need to know, instead of what I want to hear. I was more blessed than lucky to have her in my life. It is so heartwarming to know that you have someone who cares so much about your well-being and is always there for you, for the good times and bad. Having a friend who also acts like an older sister is a pure treasure; a real gem. Lita has been a pillar of support during those difficult times of my life. She is more than just a friend to me, but a sister, a family. I was adopted by their family and they became part of my life for almost four decades. Lita's mother had been a mother to me; she treated me exactly as she treated her children [Lita and her siblings]. That's why, when Nana died it was very difficult for me; like losing a mother for the second time.

We were just commemorating Nana's first death anniversary, on October 10, 2010, when a month later, Lita started complaining of not feeling well. She looked haggard; exhausted and worn out. I told her to go see the doctor to find out what it is, reminding her what happened to Nana. Moreover, five years ago she had surgery at Princess Margaret Hospital on her right breast because of the pus discharge from her breast, and later diagnosed as papilloma - It had been biopsied, but it was benign. However, she was advised to have it checked every six months but never did.

One morning, I was about to go to work when I heard her crying upstairs. I went over what was wrong with her. When I opened the door, I saw her holding her head.

"What's wrong with you?" I was concerned.

"I had a terrible headache!" she replied.

I was alarmed because when I looked at her, she had a flushed face. I took her blood pressure and it was registered to 198/100 mmHg

"OMG! Your blood pressure is very high!" I exclaimed.

"I don't know why?" she uttered in pain.

"Let's go to the hospital to have it checked, you don't know what triggered your blood pressure to go up like that!" I announced.

"No, I don't want to go to the hospital. Just give me Tylenol, maybe when my headache disappears I will feel better," she reasoned out.

I gave her two tablets of Tylenols and chamomile tea to drink; put a warm compress on her forehead and asked her to relax and do deep breathing exercises. I asked her to lay down on her left side, to relieve pressure on the blood vessels that return blood to heart. These vessels are located on the right side of the body and can be compressed by slowing its circulation if you sleep on your right side. After half an hour I went back to take her BP again, and was relieved that it went down a lot - 152/90 mmHg. It's still high, but much better than it was.

"How are you feeling now?" I asked.

"Much better. I have pain on my right breast though," she said anxiously.

I touched the area where she was complaining of pain. I was frightened because I felt the lump there. It's big!

"You have to make an appointment to see your doctor tomorrow, or I will take you to the hospital now," I told her in a serious voice.

She knew me better, that I will do as I said I am going to do. She called her doctor and made an appointment to see him the following day.

After her GP examined her, it was confirmed that there was a lump indeed. He gave her a requisition for mammogram and ultrasound ASAP. She went to the Medical Lab near us. After two weeks, I was home when the phone rang. It was the Lab - looking for her. I told her that I am Lita's sister and I want to know the result of her Mammogram and ultrasound. She declined because of 'confidentiality' as Per se. I gave Lita's number at work. In the meantime, I was terrified, thinking the worst ahead. I can feel it in my guts that something bad is going to happen. When she came home I anxiously asked if she spoke to the Radiologist.

"Yes, she called me at work," she said dejectedly.

"and…what is it?" I asked, afraid to hear what's coming.

"There is a lump there. The Radiologist wanted to repeat the mammogram and to do the CT scan as well, to make sure not to miss anything," she explained.

"So, did you book an appointment?" I tried to compose myself.

"Not yet! I will do that on my day off." She replied.

Lita is an extremely dedicated and committed employee. She has a near- perfect attendance; never call-in sick even when she was not feeling well. She is always going above and beyond what is expected to do and is really taking on the mantle of the ideal employee. She always put her job as her priority over her health which pissed me off sometimes.

"Are you in denial? They found a lump in your breast, I felt it too, it's huge! And you're telling me that you are going to wait for your day off to do what's requested of you. It's insane! You think your work will put a statue of you when you're six feet under the ground? You call and book an appointment for your mammogram and CT scan ASAP, now at this very minute and call- in sick, or else I will do it for you, myself." I was livid!

Upset with me, but she knew I was right. She went and booked an appointment at the Diagnostic and Laboratory Clinic the next day and she called her work requesting to take a day off. After 3 days the radiologist called her and she sent the result of her Mammogram, and CT scan to her GP to discuss the result with her. A few hours later, her GP's secretary called Lita to come to the clinic as the doctor would like to see her as soon as possible. The result confirmed more telling than the first one; she had a lump the size of a lime on her right breast [7.4 cm]. She is going to send her to a breast cancer specialist to find out if it is benign or cancerous through biopsy.

It was January 24,2011, when Lita received a call from the specialist to come to his office. I accompanied her to this appointment; the doctor was in his late sixties. He thoroughly examined Lita and while he was doing that, he kept asking questions about her history, any discomfort and how long the lump had been there. After he was finished, he sent Lita upstairs for a biopsy and he will call Lita after one week to discuss the result. We went upstairs for Lita to have the biopsy done, when she came out and told me that when the technician took the needle out it was bleeding, it made me even more anxious because I read somewhere that cancer cells are friable and bleed easily but I kept everything to myself as not to scare her further.

Waiting for the result is the most anxious, scary and worrying time of the whole process, whatever the outcome is. However, I kept reminding Lita that until we have the results, these are thoughts and not facts. That "we will cross the bridge when we get there", but it is easier said than done.

Less than a week later, the specialist secretary called Lita to come to his office on February 2, 2011, to discuss the biopsy's result. It coincided on Nana's birthday. I took a day off to accompany her. I bought a notebook and a pen to record everything. We got there half an hour earlier than our appointment. I can tell that Lita was very nervous and anxious, and so am I but I tried to compose myself because I need to be strong for her. A few minutes later, we were ushered into the doctor's office. We sat there for at least twenty minutes, then the door opened - it was the doctor with a stack of papers in his hand.

"Good morning! Sorry to keep you waiting. I had to review your biopsy result before I came here," he said looking at Lita.

"And what is it doctor?" I asked nervously.

"I am sorry, but the biopsy confirmed that It is indeed cancer as I had suspected. I have to explain to you the result of your biopsy: unfortunately, your cancer has advanced – stage 3, it will probably require a total mastectomy. You have what you called "Invasive Ductal Carcinoma", grade 3, HER2 positive [human epidermal receptor 2] and most likely it has spread through your lymph nodes under your armpit, at least nine or maybe more. The extent of the damage or how far it went we have no way of knowing. We just have to keep our fingers crossed that it didn't do much damage as yet. Based on your history, in 2005, you had surgically removed papilloma in your right breast, somehow it has developed into Invasive Ductal Carcinoma. The surgical Oncologist who removed your papilloma recommended for you to have it checked every six months to monitor for any cell abnormalities. However, you did not follow through with his recommendation, if you do maybe you have a different outcome than what it is now. I will send all the reports

to Princess Margaret Hospital. The Oncologist will probably contact you within the span of two weeks or so to plan the best course of treatment," he explained thoroughly.

I felt like I was in school, taking notes; writing all this information so I would not forget them. Meanwhile, Lita sat quietly, emotionless - spaced out.

"Doctor, as an expert in this field, what do you think her chances of survival of this type of cancer are?" I asked, looking him straight in the eye.

Based on the statistics of the cancer she had: IDC, HER2 positive, T3, grade 3 and N9 her survival rate is from 59% and higher, but this is just a statistic." He was forthright.

After thanking him, we left for home. Lita was very quiet while we were in the car; she just cried. I tried to console her; reassuring her that she would not travel in this difficult journey alone; I would be with her every step of the way. Other than that, nothing else I could say to make it better or ease her fear that she might die. When she got home, she ran upstairs and just screamed out crying.

"I have no one to blame but myself! I ignored the recommendation by the doctor to have it checked every six months. I brought this upon myself, now I may be going to die!" She was extremely distraught.

"I had never failed to remind you - to get it checked. However, we cannot benefit from blaming ourselves, 'what could have been or should have been'. We have to focus and put all our energy on how

78

to face and navigate in this difficult juncture of your life," I said I tried to be strong for her.

Less than a week later, Lita receives a call from Princess Margaret Hospital confirming her appointment to come to the hospital to meet with the Oncologist, surgical oncologist, social worker, dietitian, and other health team who would be involved in her care. As it was discussed by the previous specialist, it was repeated and explained to us again the type of cancer she had. We'd been told that she would have a total mastectomy on her right breast including the axillary lymph node dissection of 9 nodes and maybe more under her armpit. After the surgery, she would receive 21 rounds, or cycle of chemotherapy along with Herceptin for HER2 positive for a year. HER2 gene common to a very aggressive form of cancer like what Lita had which accounts for 20% of cases. Herceptin works by attacking itself to the HER2 receptors on the surface of breast cancer cells and blocking them from receiving growth signals. By blocking the signals, Herceptin can slow or stop the growth of breast cancer. Herceptin is an example of an immune targeted therapy developed by Dr. Dennis Slalom of UCLA. After chemo, she would do the radiation to kill the remaining cancer cells. The drugs they would use for the treatment had also been discussed, the cost – which would be paid by her private insurance at work and the rest would be paid by OHIP [Ontario Health Insurance Plan]. Every health care provider brings in their specialties to the table to try and help Lita cope and navigate this difficult journey of her life "living with cancer". Indeed! It is going to be a long journey and winding road ahead with a lot of steep hills to climb, and an unknown path to travel. Exploring the unknown requires tolerating the uncertainty.

She had a total mastectomy of right breast on March 2,2012, and an axillary dissection. It took about two and a half hours. According to the surgical oncologist the surgery was a success; the removed twenty-one [21] lymph nodes under her armpit as "an abundance of caution". The surgery was an outpatient procedure; after she was checked and everything was okayed we were sent home. The first two nights were extremely painful; I couldn't move her arms. She can't take a shower after 48 hours as she had a drain in her incision.

The next two weeks were busy in and out of Princess Margaret Hospital – blood work, MRI, CT scan. Making sure that her body is ready to start for treatment – chemotherapy and Herceptin. The first week of chemo she was fine; no symptoms. However, after two weeks she started to really feel so sick. She was throwing up, nauseated and in extreme pain, sometimes she crawled down the floor as she had no more energy or strength to continue.

"I can't take it anymore. I have no more strength left in me to fight. Just let me go and let me die," she said crying

"No! I will not let you. I need you to fight with me. Please don't give up…it is difficult right now, but there is always hope beyond what we can see. Let's pray and ask God for strength and courage to keep going. Life is worth fighting for, we have to cling even for that little glimmer of hope," trying to encourage her.

It was extremely difficult for me to watch her in pain and suffering every single day. I want to help – take some of those loads away, but I couldn't. Sometimes, I feel guilty for pushing her to cling to life when what I saw was suffering. But I couldn't lose her, she is an integral part of my life. Honestly, I didn't know what I would do if I lost her. For more than three decades she had been my sounding board - "the wind beneath my wings". She saw me through those difficult journeys – encouraged me, prayed with me and never let go of my hand, she was the wind beyond my sails. She is more than a friend, a sister, she is my family in every sense of the word. Inside, I am falling apart, I am terrified of what's ahead, but I had to believe that this difficult journey will lead us to a beautiful destination.

Added to my stress, on top of dealing with Lita's illness was my work, who gave me a hard time because of the absences I was taking to accompany Lita to all her appointments, including chemo and laboratories. But I cannot afford to falter; I need to be strong for her, as I promised Nana.

She was on her third week of chemo when we were informed that she couldn't have the treatment that day because her liver enzyme was very high.

"What now?" I thought to myself.

The following week, she had blood work done and we were directed to see the oncologist to discuss the blood result.

"Good morning! I am sorry, but we have to stop the chemotherapy because your liver enzyme reached the level which is extremely concerning. It could risk the liver to fail if we continue the treatment. I referred your case to a hepatologist, and she suggested for Ms. Tumbaga to have a scan on your liver to see what's going on there. Then she wants to have the liver biopsy for abundance of caution because of the symptoms

she was exhibiting: jaundice and abdominal pain," she explained thoroughly

"How long until we find out the result of the CT scan and the biopsy? What happened to her treatment doctor?" I asked with concern.

"The treatment will continue, but for now we have to temporarily stop it until we find out what's causing the liver enzyme to reach a staggering almost a thousand. I will call you once I have all the results," she replied.

We went home extremely disappointed and beaten up – physically and emotionally exhausted. Cancer is like a teeter-totter – it brings you up, then drops you down.

I spent the whole night searching on the internet, I think I visited all the sites looking for alternative medicines to help bring down Lita's liver enzyme level. I stumbled upon something which I thought was worth trying. It is, according to the author, extremely powerful to detox the liver from toxins caused by foreign substances – like chemo drugs. The formulas are: 10 garlic globes, 1 tbsp of turmeric, 1 tbsp of Oregano, 1 root of beets, 1 red onion, 1 large carrot. Bring to a boil, then simmer and let her drink it – serve as her water. For breakfast, I made her all the berries smoothie [strawberry, blueberries, raspberry, blackberry]. I went out to buy her a good juicer machine. Made her green juice first thing in the morning: 1 green apple, 1 stalk of celery, bunch of kale, and ginger root. All of these have to be organic, which cost an arm and a leg; everybody knows how expensive organic foods are. I had to go to Ambrosia to get all these organic fruits and vegetables.

After one week the oncologist called and we breathed a sigh of relief when she told us that the biopsy result was negative. The scan showed inflammation on the liver. They determined that the chemo drugs were probably the culprit for the liver enzyme to shoot high; very strong on the liver to take. Lita's oncologist told us that they had to change the chemo drug to the one that would be easier on the liver. Likewise, we were told that Lita has to rest for another two weeks, then do the lab prior to seeing her oncologist. If her liver enzyme brings to a level that is safe to continue the treatment, then she would start her chemotherapy again.

The day before her chemo schedule, we were at the hospital early in the morning for her blood work. The earlier the better because it is not as busy; fewer people. We proceeded to see her oncologist to find out if she will resume her treatment.

"Good morning! I have some good news. Your liver enzyme is back to normal. I don't know what you did, but whatever it is, continue doing it as it seemed to be working. I am pleased with the blood result," she said. It was encouraging.

"Thank you doctor! So, can I start my chemo treatment tomorrow?" Lita asked.

"Yes, with the new drug. We have to start all over again-21 cycles of chemotherapy and one year of Herceptin. Nothing has changed, except that we are using a new drug which is much easier on your liver," she explained.

"How about the side effects and the effectiveness of this new drug?" I queried.

"Every person experience chemotherapy differently, both physically and emotionally. Each person experiences side effects from chemotherapy differently, and different chemotherapy drugs cause different side effects. Many people feel fine for the first few hours following chemotherapy. Usually, some reaction occurs about four to six hours later. However, some people don't react until 12 or even 24 hours to 48 hours after treatment. Some people experience almost all of the side effects while others experience almost none. When it comes to the effectiveness of this drug, we don't know yet until after a few months of treatment if Ms. Tumbaga is responding to the treatment," she patiently explained.

Lita started her chemotherapy with this new drug. After a couple of weeks her hair started to fall off. She was weaker every session of her chemotherapy, as she had all the symptoms: nausea and vomiting, itchy and dry skin, sore mouth, diarrhea and weakness and pain on her right arm - side effect of the axillary lymph node dissection. It was a difficult journey with a lot of ups and down – navigating the challenges that arise is one way of coping with it. To varying degrees, people with cancer struggle with the challenges of coping and adjusting to these life changes. Sometimes, the chemotherapy schedules are either delayed or canceled because of different factors: whether her hemoglobin or neutrophils are low which puts her at a high risk if the treatment continues. Furthermore, every time she looked at herself in the mirror she got depressed and cried as said in the quote," she looks like a clown"; bald head and with one breast.

The physical and emotional demands of caring for loved ones with cancer can be very exhausting and even lead to burnout. But I couldn't afford to fall apart as Lita needs me more than ever. There is no one else; she doesn't have any family and relatives here except Janet and Libeth. Her other sibling lives in the state.

Finally, after a long and difficult journey she finished her chemotherapy and Herceptin. After two weeks, she started with her radiation therapy – 5 days a week [Monday to Friday] for seven weeks. For almost a year and a half, our lives evolved between home and hospital: treatments, doctors' appointments, laboratories, and imaging [ultrasound, CT scan, MRI]. Sometimes I wonder, if you survive the cancer most likely you are going to get another form of cancer from the radiation you get your body exposed to.

Lita completed all her treatment, in spite of many difficult challenges. The nurses at the chemo wards were ecstatic for her and wished her good luck for her next endeavor to fight this evil disease. We went to see her oncologist the week after.

"Congratulations, you did it! So far so good, your laboratory results are good. We will wait for three months before you will have a complete CT scan to determine if you responded to the treatment. In the meantime, try to go back to living your life Ms. Tumbaga. Don't let cancer deprive or rob you of happiness in living your life to the fullest," she said emphatically.

"Thank you very much for all your help and patience towards me over the course of my treatment and difficult journey fighting this cancer," Lita uttered in tears.

"I echo Lita's sentiments doctor, Thank you!" I said with all sincerity.

"The pleasure is all mine. You are a very good patient Ms. Tumbaga. See you in three months and I hope by that time I have good news to tell you," she said smiling.

After three months she had her CT scan and we were elated, when Lita's oncologist told us that there is no trace of cancer in her body. She embraced her doctors delighted by the news that after a long and difficult journey she survived cancer. Although, we were told that she is not out of the woods yet because in a lot of cases cancer comes back after a year or so. But if she survives after five years, her chances of survivorship from cancer are much better. She was told to continue monitoring it by doing a CT scan every six months.

Amazingly through God's grace it's been eleven years since she was diagnosed. Lita went back to work and picked up the pieces of her life that had been distracted by cancer. There are some times, she still worries that cancer might come back, but her faith in God helped her get to the other side. She refused to let cancer define her- she believes that it's not enough that you survive this evil disease, but also to thrive and live your life to the fullest and appreciate everything in front of you. "What matters is not what happened to us, but how we react to what happened to us is more important and significant." -LFP

Lilibeth [described in chapter 6]

She was diagnosed of Colon cancer, stage 3

It's been over five years since she was been diagnosed of colon cancer.

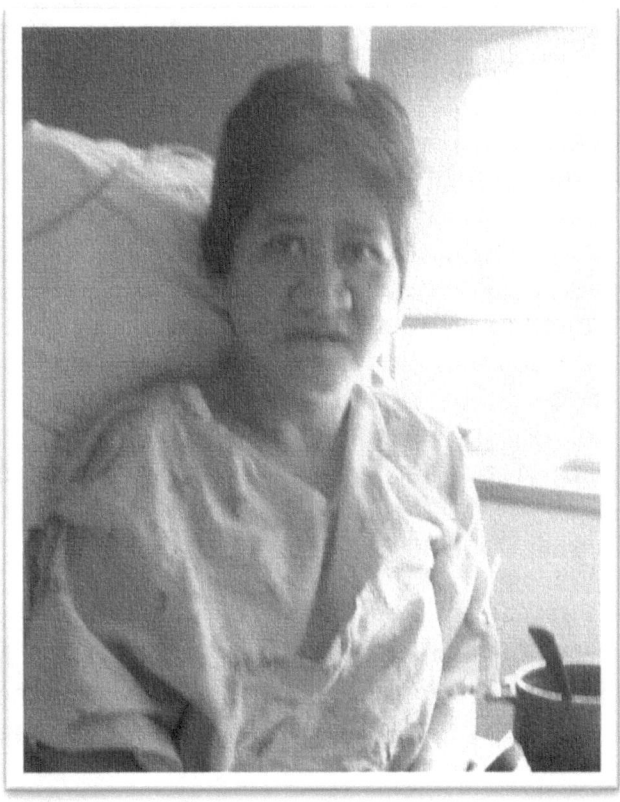

Chapter 6

So innocent to understand

Have you ever known anyone that has either experienced cancer first hand or a caregiver to someone with cancer? Chances are the answer to that is yes, and it has become painfully crystal clear that at least one in every three individuals has cancer or knows someone with cancer.

Some people might probably think that is a very high percentage, very unlikely to be true, and difficult to believe: farfetched.

However, would you believe it, if I told you that it is true! I can attest to this because I was a primary caregiver of three people in the family that had been diagnosed with cancer in just a span of seven years. First, Nana [the mother] who was diagnosed with Ovarian cancer. Then, a year later after Nana's first year death anniversary, Lita [the eldest] daughter was diagnosed with breast cancer. And after five years, Libeth [the youngest daughter] was also diagnosed with Colon cancer. Out of these three people in the family, the two daughters have survived. Nana, on the other hand, lived for almost three years after she was diagnosed; unfortunately, she succumbed to her death thereafter.

It was spring of 2017 when one evening I received a call from Lita, telling me the bad news that Libeth had passed a lot of fresh blood from her bowel. I can hear the panic and anxiety in her voice.

"Just calm down! Is this the first time that has happened? I queried, trying to calm her down.

"I don't know. She just called me this evening to show me the blood on the toilet after she finished pooping. It was a lot," she said, frightened.

"Take her to the emergency right away, because we don't know what causes the bleeding. Remember Nana?" Reminding her exactly what happened to Nana.

"Okay, I am going to take her to the hospital now. I am scared of what they might find out. I wished that you were here with me," she said worriedly.

"I wish too, but I can't leave Miriam [at the time I was working full time, right after I took an early retirement at work], and it's too late to call her daughter to relieve me. Call me as soon as you have the news, or she will be seen by the doctor. I will be waiting for a call from you," I said, trying to boost her spirit.

Waiting for news from Lita, I feel particularly ridden with anxiety during a period of uncertainty. I was overcome with sadness thinking about Libeth. Her mental capacity would not understand these things. I sat on the couch quietly asking God, *"why?"*.

"Am I going to go through with this again?" I was furious asking God.

Come to think of it, it's really inconceivable that three people in the family [although, Libeth not confirmed yet] would be touched with cancer. It's really appalling.

My cell phone rang and it was Lita, crying uncontrollably. It took me a while to calm her down and for her to tell me what was the result of all the tests done with Libeth.

"It was confirmed she has cancer! The doctor that took the colonoscopy just left. He explained that Libeth had colon cancer," she said in great anguish.

"Did they tell you how bad it is?" I asked dejected

"No! And I didn't ask. I was so overwhelmed by the news that I was not thinking clearly. Why did it happen to us? First Nana, then me, now Libeth! It is too much to bear," she said in distraught voice.

"Did you have the name of the doctor, who performed the colonoscopy? How was Libeth now, did she know what's going on?" I asked anxiously.

"Yes, he left the number to call him to arrange a meeting with the oncologist and the surgeon. Libeth is here, she is crying. Asking a lot of questions, although when I told her she didn't understand. She just kept asking me if she is going to die like Nana," Lita said crying again.

"Okay, if you're done there now, take Libeth home. I know this news about her having cancer is horrifying. But we will pass through it, like what we did before. You have to try to be strong for her and you must not forget that you just recovered from the disease yourself. Stress is definitely not good for you. I will ask Miriam's daughter if she could stay with Miriam even just for a couple of hours so that I can come home and get all the information. I will handle everything from here on," reassuring Lita that she is not alone.

After I hung up the phone, I sat on the couch still in shock by the news of Libeth being diagnosed with cancer. I promised Nana that I am going to look after them, and I will do exactly that. It is extremely upsetting news, and very hard to take those three members of the family diagnosed with cancer? However, no matter how distressing this new turn of events, we have no choice but to face it head on. I had to be strong for all of us.

I called my client's daughter - asking a huge favor if I can go home for even just a couple of hours to see my family, to be with them in this difficult situation. After I explained the reasons why she definitely understood. She told me to take a whole day to be with my family - they may not be my blood family, but they've been my family in every sense of the word.

When I got home I found Libeth crying upstairs. She may not understand the whole thing about her disease, but she knew it's very bad - that she could die, like Nana. I tried to comfort her, promising that I would take care of her, like I took care of Nana and Lita. Life is really unfair! Why Libeth? She is so innocent to understand what's going on? She may be fifty years old but her mental capacity is just similar to a five-year-old kid. I spent time comforting her and explaining to her about her disease - not all people that had been diagnosed with cancer will die, some people survived too, like Lita, her sister. Once she calmed down, I took all the information from Lita and left for work.

The next day, I called this doctor, the gastroenterologist who performed the colonoscopy on Libeth. I left messages, upon messages but I didn't get a reply yet. What I learned from experience dealing with these doctors, sometimes you need to be a pest, nagging them all the time to get an answer. After three days, finally he called me back.

"Hi, I am Doctor Y, sorry for not being able to get back to you quickly. I was away for a conference and I just got back today, and according to my secretary you've been calling about your sister Lilibeth Tumbaga. Yes, it had revealed that she had colon cancer after I performed the colonoscopy. The tumor was at the bottom of her colon - very close to the Vagina. It's huge, and it's already almost the end of stage 3. Our worry, the tumor that big could have spread to the liver. That's why we needed to have a scan on the liver and a

complete CT scan on the abdomen to make sure that it hasn't spread to the surrounding area. And most likely, they have to shrink the tumor before the surgery and may be followed by radiation therapy. But that's for the oncologist and the surgical oncology to decide. I had sent out all the information to Doctor P [surgeon] and Doctor T [oncologist]. You have to call them to arrange an appointment to discuss the best possible treatment option," he explained thoroughly.

"Thank you so much Doctor Y for that detailed information, and I am sorry if I was a pest; just that I am worried about my sister's condition and as you know she is a mentally challenged. Knowing full well what we are up against will give me more options on how to navigate in handling my sister and the best way to help her," I said, grateful to Doctor Y.

After I hung up the phone on Doctor Y, I did not waste any time. I called both the oncologist and the general surgeon in-charge of Libeth's care to arrange a meeting with both of them to discuss the best course of treatment for Libeth. The next day, Doctor T called me back and she sounded very nice and patient in answering all my questions. She agreed with Doctor Y to do the scan on the liver and MRI on the whole abdomen to make sure that the cancer had not spread yet to the neighboring organ or tissues. I have to pick up the requisition from her clinic, then take Libeth to the imaging department to have the CTScan and MRI done. Then, both of them are going to meet with us after two weeks. To discuss the possible treatment for Libeth. I felt a sigh of relief after I had spoken to these doctors - the oncologist and the general surgeon. All my questions had been answered by them.

Now, I had to focus on Libeth treatment to start as quickly as it could, for cancer is not waiting, sleeping until the doctors are ready to start the treatment.

I felt so bad to ask my client's daughter again for a day off but I had no choice, I had to take care of Libeth. I could not leave it to Lita, as I was afraid that stress might trigger her cancer to come back. I was extremely fortunate because I had a very understanding employer, not to mention supportive. They told me that *"I have to take care of my family - they have to come first"* Truly amazing people!

I picked up Libeth from home, Janet came with us to have her CTScan and MRI done for it to be ready when we see Doctor P [general surgeon] and Doctor T [oncologist] in two weeks. While we were waiting for Libeth's name to be called for the procedure. I saw Janet crying [Libeth's older sister].

"*Are you okay Janet?*" I asked.

"*Is there really God?*" She asked in tears.

"*Of course, there is! Yes a lot of things don't make sense, we are upset because of what's happening and a lot of it we don't understand, but God's way is beyond measure, beyond understanding. As tumultuous the storms that we are walking right now, we have to believe that He will lead us to a safer ground. So, just hang on Janet, don't let go of your faith. You need to be strong, we all need to be strong for Libeth and for Lita,*" trying to comfort Janet.

Libeth had her CTScan and MRI done, after I dropped them at the house, I proceeded to my work. From time to time, Lita would call me to speak to Libeth when Libeth was throwing her tantrum, especially when she is in pain. She starts to panic and right away she thinks that she is going to die. It is extremely difficult to explain to someone that lacks the capacity to understand the whole thing. But after I spoke to her she calmed down. She listens to me, or I'd say she is afraid of me.

The day we had to meet the doctors; I went to visit Nana at the cemetery.

"Nana, I don't have to tell you what's going on, because I am sure you already know. We have to meet the doctors in charge of Libeth treatment - to explain to us the best course of treatment for her. The treatment she is going to receive is going to be based on the result of CTScan and MRI in which we are hoping and praying that it hasn't spread yet. Please Nana, put a good word to the Big guy up there to take it easy on us. I need all the help I can get, for me to carry on this task that you have entrusted to me. I have so much on my plate, but I will try to be strong for both Lita, Janet and Libeth. I will take care of them as I had promised you I would. We miss you terribly, but I know you are happy where you are now. Just keep an eye on us and guide us in our daily undertakings," spending a quiet time with Nana.

From the cemetery I picked up Libeth, then we headed to Markham Stouffville Hospital to meet the doctor. It is only about a 5-minute drive. When we got there, we were ushered by the receptionist to the doctor's office where we found the two doctors waiting for us with a stack of papers and a laptop in front of them.

"Good morning, to both of you. My name is Loretta, and I am a sister of Libeth Tumbaga. I hope we're not late." I Introduced myself and shook their hands then, I sat down.

"Good morning to both of you! And we assumed this is Lilibeth? How are you doing?" They both asked Libeth.

Libeth did not answer them, but that's the way she is, if she doesn't know you, she won't talk to you. She looked away - avoiding their eyes. I sat her down beside me, and explained to both doctors that she doesn't talk to strangers. Of course, they knew too that she is a mentally challenged. They stood up and introduced themselves to us.

"My name is Doctor T and this is Doctor P [acknowledging the woman standing beside her]. Doctor P is a general surgeon and she will perform the surgery on Lilibeth. I am one of the oncologists here at Markham Stouffville Hospital. I will be in charge of Lilibeth cancer treatment. I had a lengthy conversation with Doctor Y along with Doctor P on what the best way we can proceed to treat Lilibeth's cancer. We have good news and bad news for you. Which one would you like me to discuss first?" She asked, looking me in the eye.

"I think it would be nice to start with the good news," I said with a smile.

"Okay then, the reason that we requested for a CTScan for the liver and Complete MRI of the abdomen is to make sure that the cancer didn't invade the neighboring organs or tissues. The good news, both CTScan and MRI were turned out to be negative. However, there is bad news - the tumor is quite big so we may cut a big portion of the colon and sever a portion of her private part. So that means there is a possibility that she may wear an ostomy bag, and a possibility that when she poops it might pass through her private part. We are trying to avoid this scenario, so, therefore Doctor Y, me and Doctor P are in agreement that we will give Lilibeth a chemo pill for two months, hoping to shrink the tumor before the surgery to avoid the complication I had mentioned before. Then, after surgery she will have radiation for a month - every day. Hopefully she will respond to treatment.

Do you have any questions or concerns?" Doctor T asked while Doctor P was nodding.

"I am grateful that the cancer has not spread yet, however, I am concerned about the ostomy bag and the possibility of severing her private part. As you were all aware that she doesn't have the mental capacity to care for herself. So, hopefully the chemo pill would shrink her tumor before surgery to avoid all the complications. How about side effects Doctor?" I queried.

"She is going to take 5 - Fluorouracil or Adrucil 5 - FU every day for two months. Generally speaking, the side effects of these drugs are not that severe compared to other chemo pills but then again, every person is different," she remarked.

"Do you have any questions for me, Miss Pilatan? Doctor P asked.

"So, after two months of my sister's taking the chemo pill, are you going to do the surgery right away, or does she have to wait. After the surgery, how long does she have to stay in the hospital?" I asked curiously.

"After she finishes taking her chemo pills, we will do another CTScan to see if the cancer shrinks before the surgery. If everything goes well, according to plan, then I will proceed with the surgery, my secretary will contact you to schedule the surgery. She does not need or require to stay in the hospital, maybe just overnight to monitor her, then she is good to go home, unless there is a complication," Doctor P answered in detail.

"When is she going to start the chemo pill?" I asked.

"Today, she can start taking it. I will give you a prescription along with instructions on how to take it

96

and also the list of side effects and what to do," Doctor T replied.

The meeting was very productive. I thanked both doctors for their patience in explaining to us what we're up against and the best course of treatment for Libeth. I hope that the chemo pill will be able to shrink the tumor to prevent the anticipated complication. After I dropped Libeth home I headed back to my work. Driving alone in the car, I am leery about the possibility of her wearing an ostomy bag or severing a portion of her private part as it would be very difficult for her to manage because of her mental capacity to care for herself. However, I've learned from past experiences that worrying about what lies ahead is unproductive. I always used the phrase *"I cross the bridge when I get there".* Worrying about something that I have no control over is a waste of time and energy. I would rather spend my time and energy on the tasks at hand - the present problem.

Libeth had finished taking her chemo pills with minimal side effects [diarrhea, itchy and dry skin and a sore mouth], and of course pain. Whenever she encountered these symptoms she threw tantrums because she didn't understand that she had cancer and that she is on treatment and these symptoms are one of the side effects that she has to go through. I took her to have her CTScan done and Doctor T will notify me once she has the result. After one week I received a call from Doctor T's secretary that the result was in and Doctor T wanted to see me to discuss it. I went to see her and I was elated when she told me that the cancer has shrunk significantly and the surgery will go ahead as planned.

After a little bit more than five hours, Doctor T came to talk to us [Lita, Janet and me], to give us the good news that the surgery was a success. The tumor has shrunk so much that she was able to cut the colon with cancer and reattached it without significant damage to the colon which could result in Libeth wearing an ostomy bag. She was also able to avoid cutting a part of her vagina, so all the complications that were discussed before had been avoided. She gave us a bunch of papers for post-surgery care. Doctor P told us to make an appointment to see Doctor T and follow-up appointment to see her in two weeks. I stayed with Libeth over the hospital for the night. She was miserable complaining of pain and among other things. The next day, after she was checked by the nurse and everything seemed to be okay, she was discharged home.

After two weeks we went to see the surgeon and we were delighted to hear that Libeth's wound is healing beautifully. After seeing her, we went to see the oncologist, Doctor T and we were told that Libeth can start her radiation therapy the following week. The only downside is that, is not going to be at Markham Stouffville Hospital. It's going to be in New Market - quite a distance from where we live; half an hour drive. The radiation is every day for one month. All of us are working full time, how are we going to make it work? I can't take her every day, as my client had already given me a lot of time off during those doctor's and imaging appointments and during Libeth's surgery. I would be taking advantage of their generosity if I would ask for more time off. I spoke to Lita if she could request for a couple of weeks' vacation from work, and so is Janet, and I can pitch in here and there in between them. But I told them that I am going to take Libeth on her first radiation. So, it has been agreed between the three of us, that's what we are going to do.

It was a difficult journey, but finally, Libeth had finished her Radiation therapy with a minimal side effect [diarrhea, dry and itchy skin]. After her radiation therapy was finished, we were told that she needs to continue doing the follow-up for the next 5 years: She has to do colonoscopy every year, CTScan, Ultrasound and blood work for the next five years. It's been more than 5 years since she was diagnosed, and so far so good. It's been a difficult journey throughout, but still thankful to God that we are able to overcome the many highways and bi-ways of life living with cancer.

Neil [described in chapter 7]

Diagnosed of Diffused Large B-Cell Lymphoma

seventeen years old, who courageously, fought the cancer, unfortunately died after less than 5 months of having been diagnosed.

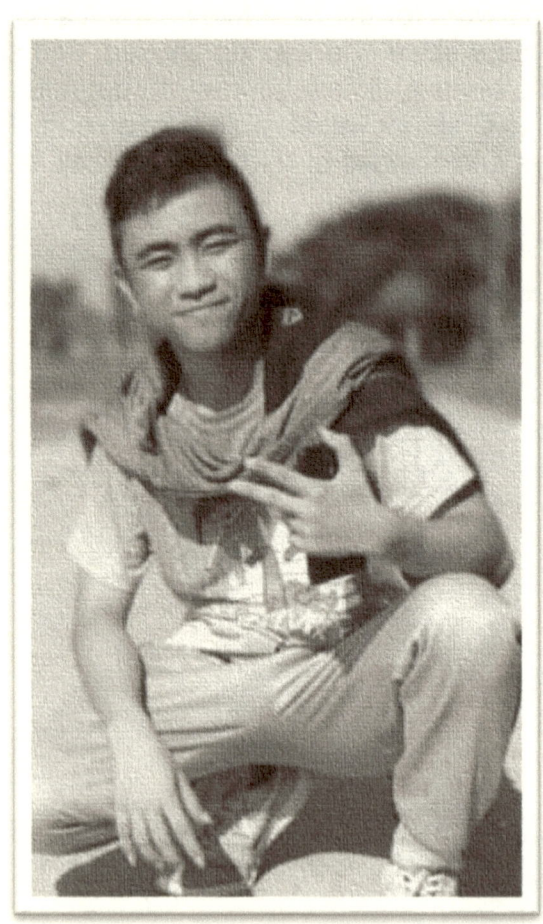

Chapter 7

Too young to die

Alberto and Nelly lived in the Philippines. They had been married for a few years but not lucky to have children of their own. Alberto is a rent farmer and Nelly is just a plain housewife, but sometimes helped her husband with work at the farm.

A distant relative was pregnant and wanted to abort the baby as they had no means to take care of another child on the way as the family had barely enough to scrape a living. When Nelly heard the news, she went to see this relative to convince her not to abort the baby, she could give them the baby instead. The relative had agreed to carry the baby full term then, will hand over the baby to Nelly and Alberto once the baby is born. She doesn't want to take the baby home with her to avoid emotional attachment. It made Nelly and Alberto elated with excitement that alas they will have a baby of their own.

When the baby was born, Nelly had asked the doctor to put them as the baby's parent [at the time adoption was simple; not complicated as it is now], so as requested this cute newborn baby boy's parents were Nelly and Alberto Lorea appeared in his birth certificate. They name him, Neil Albert Lorea, from the combination of their name – Nelly and Alberto.

According to Nelly and Alberto, Neil was a sickly child; for some unknown reason he had what you called it a "baby reflux"; he gets sick during and after feeding and regurgitates the milk. However, when he turned a year old, the symptoms had slowly disappeared. They loved this boy so much that they both tried their best to provide him with all his needs, in spite of Alberto's meager income on the farm. He was the apple of their eye; their joy and happiness. They both believed that Neil was a blessing from God given to them.

"The day God placed you into our hands, you were born into our hearts in a very special way. We prayed for you, we dreamed of you, we prepared for you, we waited for you. And when we finally held you for the very first time it felt like you'd belonged to us forever. You may not have our eyes, or our smile, but from that very first movement, you have our hearts." Nelly and Alberto simply adored their baby boy!

Neil was a good child growing up; he was loving and affectionate to his parents. He never gets himself in trouble, he does what he was told, in another word, he was almost a perfect child.

When he is old enough to understand, Nelly and Alberto have decided to tell him the truth that he is adopted. There isn't a right time to tell him that he is adopted but they thought it's best to tell him as early as possible. They don't want him learning his adoption from anyone else. They, likewise, told him who his biological parents were. He was silent for a minute or two.

"Why did they give me away?" he asked, bewildered and somewhat hurt.

But after Nelly and Alberto had explained to him the reason why, he understood.

"Neil, we may not be your biological parents, but that being adopted does not mean we love you less. The day you came into our lives, is the happiest moment of our lives. Your mom and I love you so much," they both reassured him.

"I love you both too! I am lucky that you are my parents" he replied.

As the years went by, Neil has grown to be a nice-looking young man. He never mingled himself with the wrong kind of friend. He is a very studious and responsible young man. He was a consistent honor student – from grade one to grade eleven. Nelly and Alberto had high hopes that their only child would one day become successful.

However, on May 28,2021, he was taken ill; fresh blood passed through his bowel when he tried to have a bowel movement. His parents took him to a nearby hospital – Pototan Provincial Hospital, Pototan, Iloilo. He was admitted there for further investigation and observation for *"profuse bloody stool"*. Proctosigmoidoscopy was done and the result was negative. Merckel's diverticulum scan was also done to rule out Merckel's diverticulosis for it is the most common congenital defect of the gastrointestinal tract which affects about 2% to 3% of the general population but the most common cause of bleeding in Neil's age group. The result has also turned out negative. After a blood transfusion of 4 units of blood he was discharged on June 14, 2021, with the instruction that he will be admitted to West Visayas University Hospital [Benito], a government run hospital for colonoscopy. Since the bleeding stopped, they delayed the colonoscopy until June 20, 2021. Nevertheless, another episode of bleeding recurred and his parents were in a panicky mood, overwhelmed with the sudden turn of Neil's health – they simply did not know what to do. Alberto called her second cousin, who is a well-respected in the medical community and attending physician at Mission Hospital.

"Inday, Neil was bleeding again, we don't know what to do? Please help us!" He begged his cousin in tears.

"You should take him to New Lucena Polytechnic Hospital for IV fluid to be given immediately to prevent dehydration and for him to be given medication ASAP." She strongly recommended it.

Referral to Iloilo Mission Hospital was facilitated by her [Dr. Rosalinda Palmares]. Neil was admitted at Iloilo Mission Hospital on June 20, 2021. Upper GI endoscopy was done on June 24, 2021, the result was normal. Colonoscopy was also done, in which positive for Nodular lesion with pinkish erythematous color over the distal ileum. Specimen sent to histopathology to help provide the diagnosis. On July 5, 2021, histopathology officially released the result of the specimen done, along with the immunohistology test. The result was "Diffuse Large B-Cell Lymphoma, or DLBCL.

Diffuse Large B-Cell Lymphoma is a type of blood cancer that develops when white blood cells called lymphocytes grow abnormally. Lymphocytes are part of the immune system. They travel around your body in your lymphatic system and help to fight infections. There are two types of lymphocytes: T lymphocyte [T Cells] and B lymphocyte [B Cells]. DLBCL affects the

B Cells. There are lots of different types of lymphoma, DLBCL is the most common type of Non-Hodgkin lymphoma. It is a fast growing [high grade] lymphoma.

The exact symptoms you may experience depends on where in your body the DLBCL is. They can be very variable depending on what organs or tissues are affected. In Niels case the DLBCL must have affected his bowel.

I can't just imagine what Alberto and Nelly were feeling when the doctor had told them about Neil's diagnosis. Intense shock, confusion, disbelief, and denial. Not to mention anger and feeling bitterness and unfairness. When her cousin [Dr. Palmares] found out about the diagnosis, she rushed to their side to comfort them and as well as to explain to them what they're up against. How much of these they understand.

"Alberto, Nelly, Neil, I am so sorry about this bad news. Do you guys understand what this means?" She asked them with great concern and empathy.

"Not really, 'Inday'. I was overwhelmed with shock and so much information that I cannot process it in my head. The only thing I understood was that Neil had cancer," Alberto uttered crying.

"Neil had a Diffuse Large B-Cell Lymphoma, or DLBCL. It is also considered a cancer of the blood. However, Leukemia usually occurs in the bone marrow, while Neil's cancer [Lymphoma] originates in the lymphatic system and mainly targets lymph nodes and lymph tissues," she explained avoiding more complicated medical terms.

"Am I going to die Tita [auntie]?" Neil asked anxiously and sad.

"Not everyone that has cancer died. There is treatment out there, and hopefully you will respond to treatment. I am going to talk to Pediatric Oncologist in-charge of your case to discuss the course of treatment, then we'll take it from there," she said candidly.

"Thank you very much Tita, for helping and guiding us navigate this difficult journey we are facing," Neil uttered gratefully.

"Alberto, I have to be forthright with you, cancer treatment is very expensive from laboratories, imaging, treatment drugs, doctors, and hospitals. I know what your situation is; you can't afford all these things on your own. You need help from the government – NGO and other charitable organizations. I will facilitate Neil to be a "Service Patient". What it means if you qualify; You don't pay for the hospital, doctors and you get a discounted laboratory charge. However, the treatment, you have to pay from your own pocket. I could help Neil transfer to West Visayas hospital, since it is a government hospital they have more access to maybe get Neil some help for his treatment," Dr. Palmares explained comprehensively to her cousin.

"I would rather have him here at Mission Hospital [IMH] where you were working than take him at Western Visayas Medical Center [Benito] hospital. I will be lost there as I don't know anything. Everything is new to me, at least at Mission you are here to guide us on how to navigate this difficult time of our life. if I have to sell my carabao [water buffalo he used to till the land he farmed], I will for nothing more important

than to get my son help to get better," Alberto said, determined to her cousin.

"I will try my utmost best to help Neil get the help he needs to get better, but we have also to be realistic and be prepared for the worst. We need a lot of prayers and guidance from God. Keep the faith and stay positive," she encourages them.

Dr. Palmares used her connection to facilitate Neil getting in as a "Service Patient". Service Patient is a program by the hospital who has a medical training program and affiliated medical schools to help those downtrodden Filipinos who don't have the means to pay medical bills. However, only hospitals and doctors are free. You also get discount on diagnostic procedures and laboratory but you have to pay for the medicine and treatment. However, if you have no means at all to even pay for the drugs or treatment there are agencies and local governments who would help you, but you have to wait...

Since Neil was seventeen years old, he would still be under the care of a Pediatrician. Dr. Palmares had spoken to a colleague at MIH who is in charge of the Pediatric Oncologist Department, Hematology Section. The treatment for Neil was discussed. Since DLBCL can advance quickly, It has suggested that treatment must be done quickly. He was going to get a combination of chemotherapy and antibody drugs known as R-CHOP [Rituximab, Cyclophosphamide, Doxorubicin, Vincristine, and Prednisone. The R-CHOP regimen will be given in 21-day cycles [once every 21 days] for an average of 6 cycles. How quickly the medical team would start the treatment depends on the family's financial capabilities.

Alberto and Nelly sold their animal, but it was not enough to pay for the treatment. Rituximab alone cost about eighty thousand pesos per treatment, plus the chemotherapy combination drugs. They went to their local government, DSWD [Department of Social Welfare and Development]. The DSWD is a government agency mandated by law to develop, administer and implement comprehensive social welfare programs designed to uplift the living conditions and empower the disadvantaged children, youth, women, older persons, persons with disabilities, families in crises and at-risk, and etc.

The family pitched in to give whatever amount they could give to help out, including Dr. Palmares. The biological parents were also actively trying to help but they're also underprivileged. I can't just imagine how heartbreaking it is for Nelly and Alberto; it is hard enough and devastating for their only child to get cancer but it is heart wrenching to not be able to give him the help he needs to get better because of poverty, when you don't have the means!

This is where I came into the picture, or rather I came to know Neil. My sister was diagnosed with cancer back in June 2021, Dr. Palmares was my sister's attending physician. I was very active in my sister's treatment, I am in constant communication with all her medical team, including Dr. Palmares. During the course of those two months, I was awed and in admiration of how kind hearted she is - always had time for me and patiently answered all my questions about my sister's prognosis and she helped me to facilitate in finding an oncologist for my sister. We became friends.

In the meantime, my sisters were very anxious about having chemotherapy because she was afraid that she might lose her hair and she would become bald. To humor her I had my hair shaved off, then called her via video chat that she has nothing to worry because if she lost her hair she would get company - me. She chuckled and burst into laughter when she saw my bald head. She told me, "*I look like I am about to go into a "death chair"* [electric chair].

When my client's children saw my bald head, they asked me *"why?"* I told them about my sister who had been diagnosed with cancer. They gave me two thousand dollars for cancer research in my sister's name. Pondering over it, Canadians have better access to treatment than the Filipinos, so I asked them if I could donate the money instead to the Philippines cancer foundation to help those less fortunate people seeking help. They told me that I can do what I want - it's up to me.

I called Dr. Palmares if she knew any cancer organizations in Iloilo, and she recommended the Friends of Cancer Kids Iloilo Foundation. So, I sent out the money to be given to that charity. During the course of our conversation, she had mentioned that hope her nephew could avail even just five thousand pesos from that amount to help him with his treatment.

"What's wrong with your nephew Doctora?" I asked with curiosity.

"He has cancer Lori, his parents had no capacity to pay for his treatment therefore, he is still waiting for help from the government agency," she explained.

"How much will it cost for the treatment?" I queried.

"I am not sure; I will ask her pediatrician about the cost," she replied.

The following day when we talked, she told me that eighty thousand for rituximab and five thousand for chemotherapy in one treatment. Thinking about this young man made me sad; it brought back an old painful memory about my beloved niece who died of cancer at the age of only thirteen years old. I prayed to God if He wanted to use me as an instrument to help this young man to please direct me to the right person. It was the Federal election at that time; I am an active volunteer in my local riding. Somehow, I found the courage to bring the case of Neil to my local candidate. After she heard Neil's desperate need of money for his treatment, she told me she will help him; she would pay for his treatment. She asked me to pick up the money the following day so that Neil could start his treatment. Dr. Palmares couldn't be happier when she found out. I sent out the money right away, and I was ecstatic to know that Neil had his first treatment.

After a week, I got a chance to talk to him in person. He was a nice - looking young man, very bright, a bit shy but very bright. He has so much potential and a bright future ahead of him. He reminded me so much about my niece and the difficulties of not having enough money to pay or give someone you loved the best care for them to get a chance to survive and live.

"Hi, Neil, how are you feeling?" happy to see him.

"I am okay Ma'am Lori. Thank you for helping me to have my treatment. I am extremely grateful for your generosity," he said genuinely.

"Your welcome Neil. First of all, I don't want to be called Ma'am, second, it's not my money; I am just an instrument used by God because he heard your prayers for help. Please, don't lose hope, keep praying and keep hoping. Your aunt told me that you're worried about your hair that might fall off. It will grow back again. Don't worry I will send you hats and toque to cover your head. What's your favorite team?" I was delighted with this young man.

"New York, Yankees," he said shyly.

"Okay, then, I will make sure you get your Yankees hats, but why not Blue Jays? I don't like the Yankees!" I said jokingly.

I was so pleased to finally get a chance to talk to Neil. I was determined to help this young man in whatever way I could for him to get the treatment. He deserves a chance for life, to pursue his dream whatever that may be. He is too young to die yet. After his first treatment with his R-CHOP, he has to rest for 21 days before he will have the second treatment. I need to come up with another 80 thousand plus, for the second treatment- that's about 2,500 dollars Canadian. When my local politician saw me, she gave me one thousand dollars to help for the second treatment [she doesn't want her name to be mentioned], as the media might use it as propaganda to make a story.

I thought of something to fundraise money for her second treatment. My birthday was coming, so I called all my cousins and close friends, not to buy me a gift, instead to give me any amount to help pay for the treatment of this young man who has cancer in the Philippines. I have a big family here in Toronto, and I was able to fundraise enough money for Neil second treatment. I sent out the money right away to Dr. Palmares for Neils treatment. She also sent me a video of Neil wearing all those Yankees hats and toque I sent for him. The smile on his face was priceless. *"Nothing is more heartwarming to see someone smiling and you are the reason for that smile".*

Unfortunately, Neil's second round of treatment was halted because his SGPT [liver enzyme] was very high; therefore, they cannot proceed to give him the treatment as doing so could have a detrimental effect on his liver; his liver might fail. The medical team looking after him waited, and waited for his SGPT to improve but to no avail. Instead, Neil's last laboratory and Scan revealed that the cancer had advanced or metastasized. I was extremely disappointed and sad, for him and his family. However, this is life, we have to learn to accept what life throws at our path and learn to roll with the punches.

Neil asked his aunt, Dr. Palmares if he can go home and wait there for his SGPT to go down instead, as he was worried about the bill in the hospital, and maybe he feels it inside him that he is losing the battle - he just wants to go home. After consultation with his attending physician and other health team, he was discharged from Mission hospital.

Dr. Palmares, facilitated for him to get laboratory service in the house as he was so sick to travel. After a couple of weeks, he asked his father to get the result of his laboratory, then sent a message to his attending physician that he might be coming in for treatment as his father went to get the lab result. His father was about to get a tricycle to go home, when a relative, running out of breath, told him to hurry home as Neil collapsed and he was dead. He rushed home and found Neil's lifeless body in Nelly's arm, crying inconsolable.

"Alberto, our son is gone," she uttered crying.

"No, I am going to take him to the hospital, they can still revive him, you will see…" he said in denial.

Alberto, carried Neil's lifeless body to the tricycle and directed the driver to take him to a local hospital. But he was pronounced dead on arrival [DOA]. Upon hearing the word "dead" it finally sunk in that Neil was indeed gone!

Neil Albert Lorea, died just after five months of being diagnosed with cancer. A bright young man with so much potential. Like my niece, he is too young to die.

When I went home to the Philippines, I went to see them to see how they were coping with the tragic death of their son and as well as to interview them for this book and ask their permission if it is okay for me to use Neil's story. Nelly and Alberto gave me a hug with tears in their eyes.

"Ma'am Lori, Thank you for all your help to our son. We will be forever indebted to you for the rest of our life," they both said in tears.

"It was my privilege to know Neil, even though the outcome is not what I wanted to be. It must be very devastating to both of you to lose a son. Cry as much *as you can, take your time to grief, but please don't lose hope, because hope is all that we have to cling on. Keep your faith in God, and keep believing that both of you will be okay, you still have each other,"* understanding how it feels to lose a loved one.

"Thank you, but why did God give Neil to us if he is only going to take him away from us?" Nelly asked, crying.

"Trust me, Nelly I asked that same question so many times, however, there are a lot of things we don't understand how God does things, but one thing is clear, in everything that happens in our lives have a reason. We may not know it now but later it will become clear and fit like a puzzle," Speaking through experience.

I end up not able to finish the interview because I can see how it's affecting them every time Neil's name is mentioned. It brought them back to that nightmare; reliving a tragic demise of their son to cancer.

I left with a heavy heart, but like me and others that lost a loved one, they will be okay. Time will heal their wound, it might leave a deep scar, but they will be okay.

Herminia [described in chapter 8]

A retired nurse, who was diagnosed with Laryngeal or throat cancer. She was so determined to live that she fought every fiber of her being to defeat this horrible disease, but succumbed to her death after over a year since she was been diagnosed.

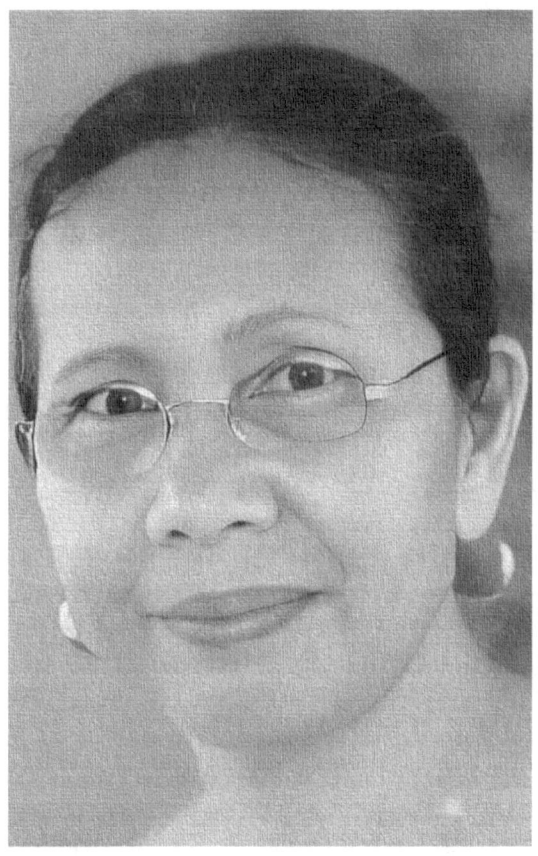

Chapter 8

Never get easy

My sister was the eldest child among eight children from the second marriage of my mother and father. She had a rocky relationship with my parents, especially my mother because she got married right after she graduated in nursing. My mother felt like she abandoned us when we needed her the most [my father went broke and my two elder brothers next to her died in a tragic death]. We were struggling to make ends meet, the reason that I had left at a young age to venture in a foreign land, to seek for a greener pasture for myself and my family.

However, after a while my mother realized that it is not my sister's job to send us to school, nor be obligated to pay my parents for her education; it is their responsibility as parents, not my sister.

Despite my sister's inability to help my parents financially, she was a very good daughter to them. When both of my parents were taken ill my sister never hesitated to take them both to her house, so she could take care of them whenever the needs arose. After my mother and father died, she took the role of making sure that we stayed close together as siblings. She would arrange Christmas dinner, New Year, and birthdays for the entire family for us to continue that sense of closeness as a family. She was present in all the births of my nephews and nieces. She was known to them as their "Mama Neng ", because that's what she was, a second mother to all them. My sister and I were alike in a lot of ways - were both outspoken; we don't mince words; we speak in a very direct and honest way without worrying about offending someone. She was very strict, but she had a good heart, very caring and doting to all her nephews and nieces. As a matter of fact, she helped our disadvantaged nieces and nephews to finish school. She would take them to her house to make sure they finished school and had their education. She strongly believed in education.

My sister had only one son, whom she adored and loved so much. When her son was just barely a year old, and she was struggling financially to make ends meet, I suggested this to her.

"Neng, why don't you apply to work abroad like our cousins and most of your friends? The salary of nurses is far more lucrative than in the Philippines. I am going to pay for your processing expenses, and surely, our cousin and your friend will not hesitate to help you find a job abroad, if you ask them," I suggested it to her.

"Bud's, I have only one son, what am I going to do with money if I were to be separated from him? I want my son to feel love and be raised by me, not raised by a stranger. I don't care even if we don't have enough money as long as we are together as a family," she said with all conviction.

Since then, I never bring up the subject again. But my mother from time to time would express disappointment; she thought that my sister just wasted her education and had no ambition at all.

"We sent you to school so that you may have more opportunities to better your life and a brighter

future for you and your family, but instead you're not using your education. You have a Bachelor of Science degree in Nursing, far better education than other nurses that went abroad. But you have opted, instead, with your meager income as a Public Health Nurse, to stay here rather than working abroad to secure a richer future for your son and your family." My mother gave my sister an earful.

"Nay [mother], I am extremely grateful for the education you afforded me, in spite of the hardship you and Tatay had to sacrifice just for me to finish school and I am very sorry that I was not able to meet your expectation of me to help my younger sibling for their schoolings. Yes, there are plenty of opportunities awaiting me working abroad and it's true I will earn more than triple what I am earning as a Public Health Nurse. But there is more to life than merely money; my son and my family are far more important to me. They're everything to me!" my sister reiterated to my mother.

This conversation was on and off the radar between my sister and my mother. It was only put to rest when my mother died - the subject died with her.

However, my sister seemed happy and was content with her life. She loved her job as a public health nurse. My sister was very frugal; she was good with money. With her small salary as a nurse, she still managed to save up and bought a lot and later built their own house on it.

When my sister and son got married, they stayed with them, and she was extremely delighted at the birth of her first grandchild. She was the apple of my sister's eye. She would do anything for her – my sister was a very protective and a doting grandmother. Her daughter in-law was also a nurse, she applied to work for London, United Kingdom and got accepted to work in one of the long-term cares. A couple of years later, my nephew followed her. They left their four years old daughter for my sister to take care of. My nephew and his wife had another child, a baby boy in the U.K. When he was six months they brought them back to the Philippines for my sister to take care of, as it was extremely expensive to pay for a babysitter in London.

My sister raised her two grandchildren with much love and affection. She spoiled them a bit too, but I think all grandparents do. She made sure that their needs were met; financially and emotionally. My nephew and his wife had another child in the United Kingdom - another boy. They decided to keep him there.

In the beginning, things were going well as both of them were earning a decent salary. They were able to send money monthly to my sister for their children's expenses and education. Unfortunately, my nephew lost his job, and his wife's income was barely enough to support them. They were financially strapped, especially confronting the high cost of living in London. Then, covid came, they both had it and was locked down for two weeks in their apartment. They were unable to make ends meet, not alone to send money to my sister for their children's expenses.

My sister was a retired nurse, and receiving a decent pension monthly, but with the high cost of living, was barely enough to cover their monthly expenses, especially since both kids were in a private school. My sister tried extremely hard to meet the needs of her grandchildren, even sacrificing her own well-being, that's how much she loved those kids.

My sister's life has been battered from one misfortune after another. First, she had Osteonecrosis of the femur [a condition caused by a compromise of the blood supply of the femoral head]. It was so bad that the femur bone had to be replaced, or else she would not be able to walk. It was during that time when she went through a series of tests that it revealed that she had a bone TB [is a condition when tuberculosis spreads beyond the lungs and creeps into the bones]. Then a year later, they had a serious car accident, in which her grandson and her were hospitalized, the car was in total wrecked. After a series of tests, UK [grandson, pet name after United Kingdom], was released from the hospital, however, my sister had sustained an injury on her knees [cracked] and needed to have another surgery to repair the damage. She never was the same after that; she could bear weight, and can only walk a very short distance. That was a huge blow to her independence and her quality of life.

I love my sister, but we are no different than that of other families. It came at a time that things happened which crippled the relationship. Conflict can happen when each has different views or beliefs that clash and sometimes can occur when one misunderstands each other and jumps to the wrong conclusion. In other words, my sister and I had a falling out – I did not talk to her for at least three years - just decided to temporarily exit and give us a break! Sometimes, it is easier to run away from the problem, rather than face them. So, that's what happened. I became disinterested when it came to her. I was at work, one day when my sister [here in Canada] phoned me.

"Neneng, was in the hospital at Mission. She was admitted last night because she had difficulty breathing. Please, help her - they need cash. I can't send money right now as I am running short. Call Ryan [our nephew], as he was the one who took her to the hospital," she furthered added.

"Why me? She has a son in London, he is the one that you should be talking to, instead of me," I retorted.

"Where are they going to get the money? Jonelle still doesn't have a permanent job; just part-time, part-time here and there. They're on the bread line," she replied.

"Sorry but I didn't have the money either," I said harshly.

"It's up to you, what you want to do with the information I provided." She hangs up the phone, annoyed with me.

The whole day, I had been thinking about my sister, what was wrong with her? To ease my mind, I called my nephew Ryan.

"Ryan, what's wrong with your Mama Neng?" I queried.

"I took her to Mission hospital, as she was struggling to breathe. She doesn't want to come here because she said 'no money' that's why I called auntie Fe [my sister here in Canada], and MC [her granddaughter] called her mom and dad in London. Mommy [most of my nephew and nieces called me

mommy], here talk to mama Neng." He put the phone on video call.

Seeing my sister, grasping for an air to breathe, melted away all my hurts and ill feelings toward her – it has been replaced by compassion and love. She was trying to talk with tears dribbling down her cheeks.

"Neng, don't talk. Let me speak! I am so sorry for not talking to you for a while, I let my anger get the best of me. Listen, I am here now, and that's what really matters. Don't worry about the money, I will make sure you get the help you need to find out what the problem is with you. So, don't worry anymore. Concentrate on getting better – Inday Fe and I will foot the bill for your hospital, doctors and other medical expenses. I love you, Neng!" Reassuring her.

She scribbled something in the paper and let Ryan read it.

"Thank you, Bud's [short for Buday, my pet name]. I am sorry if I hurt you in any way. I am happy because we are okay now. I love you too!" I can't help myself but cry as Ryan, reading what she wrote word by word.

I gave an instruction to my nephew to call me as soon as the doctor comes to do the rounds as I want to speak directly to her about my sister's condition. I was told that her attending physician was highly recommended by Rochelle's [my nephew's wife] sister. Unfortunately, when they tried to call me I was at work and preoccupied with my client that I was not able to answer the phone. My nephew, Ryan's girlfriend, is a nurse who was able to relay and explain to me what's happening. According to her the doctor was going to perform a tracheostomy [an incision in the windpipe made to relieve an obstruction to breathing]. The doctor who was going to do the surgery was an ENT [Ear, Nose and Throat] specialist – to help my sister breathe. I was livid when my nephew told me that my sister's attending physician was rude; she yelled at her.

"Mrs. Maquiling, you are going to have surgery tomorrow," she pronounced without explaining to my sister what the procedure is all about, according to my nephew.

"I don't want to have a surgery, doctor. I am afraid," my sister nervously uttered.

"Do you want to die? Because that's what's going to happen if you refuse to have surgery!" she yelled at her and left.

When I heard that I was outraged, I asked my nephew to give me the full name of this doctor and her telephone number. I attempted several times to call her but unfortunately I was not able to connect due to poor connection, but I left a long message on her messenger.

"I am Mrs. Maquiling's sister and I heard what you did to my sister. You marched into my sister's room – rudely announced that she is to have a surgery without explaining what the surgery is for, then yelled at her. Who the hell do you think you are? Do you think it is because of your medical profession that gives you the right to treat my sister that way? My sister is going through a tough time right now. The last thing she needs is a doctor who has no clue of what it means to have compassion and empathy. You have no business

being a doctor – I can tell you that much! You're fired!!!"
I was really indignant of what she did to my sister.

She never replied to me, but at least I aired out my sentiment and displeasure towards her. Now, I have to find my sister a new attending physician [In Canada we don't need an attending physician whenever admitted in the hospital. Canada has direct admission rules: You go directly to the emergency room, then you will be interviewed by a nurse triage - what's brought you to the emergency and other health issues, take your vital signs and then help establish what kind of care patients need, ensuring the patient gets sent to the right department. After that, you will be seen by an ER doctor. Depending on your health issue, the ER doctor might order a series of tests [blood work and imaging] to determine what's wrong with the patient. If it needs to be seen by a specialist then, the ER doctor will make such a recommendation.] However, the Philippines is more complicated, shrouded by protocol and red tape.

I was talking to my brother - asking him if he knew of anyone, an attending physician for our sister.

"Yes, Dr. Palmares. She is very good; she is an internal medicine specialist," my brother announced!

"Do you have any contact number?" I Asked my brother.

"Yes, I will give you her cell number, but if you can't get hold of her try to send a message on her messenger - FB account," he furthered added.

I called Dr. Palmares a few times on her cell but no answer. I left a message to her messenger, as my brother suggested, begging her to become my sister's attending physician. I explained in my message that my sister is in a dire need of her service.

In the meantime, my sister had her tracheostomy surgery to help her breath and she could be discharged in two days. According to my nephew, Ryan, the ENT who performed the surgery removed a piece of tumor from her left vocal cord for an incision biopsy. The result would be available in two weeks or so. My sister couldn't go home on her own – she needs a nurse or a well-trained caregiver who has knowledge on how to care for tracheostomy: to suction the tracheostomy tube, clean the suction catheter to prevent infection. I posted in a few caregivers agency "Nurse wanted" for my sister, but I almost flipped over when I heard what some of them were asking - it was outrageous! In the meantime, my nephew, Ryan, was taking charge of caring for her Mama Neng along with her girlfriend, a nurse while I am looking for a permanent full-time caregiver for my sister.

Fortunately, my sister in Canada has a friend who has a cousin in the Philippines and she had mentioned that she was looking for a job. She was a well experienced caregiver; worked in a private and hospital setting. My sister gave me her contact number to call her and set up an interview.

"Hello, how are you? I am Mrs. Maquiling's sister, and I am looking for a full-time caregiver for her. She just had a tracheostomy done recently, but she was discharged from the hospital and at home recuperating. You are highly recommended by your cousin here in Canada, that you have a wide range of experience as a caregiver. Are you interested in

working for my sister?" Conducting my interview over the phone.

"Hello, ma'am! My name is Lorna, I live in Dumanggas, not far from where your sister lives. Yes, I am looking for a job as a caregiver. I looked after clients with Tracheostomies, feeding tubes, stroke and dementia. I worked at St, Paul Hospital, as a caregiver for a few years, then in a private setting in a patient's own home. I would really love to work for your sister if she chooses me," she replied.

"That's wonderful. How much is your salary expectation for a month?" Asking her.

"It's up to you ma'am," she hesitantly uttered.

"No, it's not up to me. I don't have any idea what the going rate of a caregiver in the Philippines is. Just give me a number, then I will see if we can afford it." I was being honest with her.

"You can give me 12,000 thousand a month, If it is okay with you," she announced.

"Absolutely! You know what, I will give you 12,500 a month because of your experience and I know that my sister is in a hard case due to her tracheostomy. By the way, how would you like to get paid, monthly, or bi-weekly?" Giving her an option.

"Every 15ᵗʰ and end of the month would be great ma'am," she said pleased.

"So, that's settled then. When can you start? The earlier the better, as my nephew is the one taking care of her for the time being. You may want to meet

126

my sister before you start and also for my nephew to show you around and likewise for you to familiarize her routine. You will be off on the weekend. You start Monday morning until Saturday morning. Is that okay with you?" Giving her further details.

"I have no problem ma'am. I like to be off on the weekend because I have a four years old daughter and I would like to spend some time with her on the weekend." She sounds pleased.

"There are a few things that I'd like you to be aware of before you start working for my sister: first, I don't like to be called ma'am – you may call me ate Lori, instead. Second, my sister can be very difficult at times, just try to understand where she is coming from - she is going through tough times right now; she may have cancer. She is not telling me but I know that she is scared. Third, please be open with me and feel free to discuss whenever the problem arises, and the most important of all, I want my sister to be treated with respect and dignity and I will ensure you would get the same courtesy. I am also a caregiver, so I know how it's like to deal with sick people, both mentally and physically. Is that clear to you?" I said, being candid with her.

"Thank you, ate Lori. I promise that I will try my best to understand and help her as she journeys through this difficult time. And thank you for being honest with me, don't worry if ever a problem arises, you will be the first person to know," she replied.

I breathed a sigh of relief after I was able to find my sister a caregiver. She seemed nice over the phone; I hope things will work out for my sister's sake. I video message my sister [thank God for FB], it's much easier now to communicate with your loved ones across the globe, not to mention costless.

"Neng, good morning! How do you feel this morning? You looked rather nice and vigorous. Anyway, I have good news for you, I found a full-time caregiver for you; to take care of all your needs and help you with your ADL [activity of daily living]. Her name is Lorna, she lives in Dumanggas, not far from Barotac. She will come see you tomorrow. Then she will begin her employment on Monday and will be off on Saturday morning. You will like her because she had a wide range of experiences," telling her in detail.

She scribbled in a pad, then, a minute or two later she handed it to Ryan for him to read it to me. My heart breaks whenever I see my sister doing this; I can't imagine how it's like not being able to talk to express your voice – must be awful!

"Day, thank you so much for all that you are doing for me. Sorry, that I have to give you another problem to carry, but I have no choice as you and Inday Fe are my only hope to help me with my situation." As Ryan was reading it for me, the tears started to trickle down her cheeks.

"Neng, please don't think about that, You are not a burden to me, nor to Inday Fe. We are family, and family help and support each other at whatever cost. I know you are worried about the result of the biopsy, but try not to focus so much on that. We cross that bridge when we get there. In the meantime, I want you to be positive and be hopeful. I promise you this, you will never be going through it alone, we will journey with you together whatever paths await for us to travel. We will overcome this Neng!" Encouraging her.

"Ryan, make sure that you show Lorna how to properly clean and sanitize your Mama Neng's, tracheostomy, and how to use the suction machine," giving Ryan an instruction.

"Yes, Mommy. I will stay with her for two days to train her and monitor if things are going well before I go home to Passi," Ryan reassured me.

After three weeks, Ryan and Julie [his girlfriend] went to Mission Hospital to get the result of Neneng's CT scan, and they sent me the copy right away. The result was positive; Neneng has "Squamous Cell Carcinoma". She has three [3] tan-brown, soft, irregular tissue fragments on her left vocal cord, measuring 1 cm in aggregate diameter. The report to me is vague, or nebulous because it doesn't even mention the staging. But to whom I should direct my question – she doesn't even have the attending physician yet. I got frustrated and scared for my sister. Now the hard part; how am I going to tell her? Again, as usual I have to be strong for my loved ones - I think it's kind of my role…

My prayers have been answered, because when I checked there was a message from Dr. Palmares.

"Hi ma'am Pilatan, actually Mrs. Maquiling was under my care during her surgery to replace the bone on her femur. Why what happened to her? Anyway, she can come to my clinic, Monday to Saturday from 12 [noon] to 4:00 PM." Stated on her messenger message.

I replied back telling her how appreciative I was for accepting my sister as her attending physician. To get a picture of what's going on with my sister, I sent her the biopsy report. I likewise, stated if it's okay for her to have a group chat meeting through messenger between me, my nephew, my sister and my brother-in-law with her. While I was waiting for Dr. Palmares' response, I had to take care of the difficult task ahead; telling my sister that she has cancer!

"Good morning, Lorna! How's your Mama Neng? Is everything okay there?" Talking to my sister's caregiver.

"Good morning, Ate Lori. I just finished suctioned her Trach." She replied.

"How often do you have to suction it? If she can tolerate it try not to suction it too much because the more you suction it the more it is going to irritate and could also cause some infection. Just encourage her to try and cough it up to clear the mucus or phlegm on her own," I suggested.

"That's what I was telling Mama, Ate," Lorna replied.

"Please, get Toto Boy [my brother-in-law]. I want to talk to both of them." I asked Lorna.

"Okay, Ate Lori." She went and got Toto Boy.

My brother-in-law sits beside my sister, along with Lorna, UK, Myra and Maricel [our nephew's children whom my sister adopted]. I have been in this scene a number of times but it never really gets easier.

"Neng, To Boy, the reason that I want to talk to both of you is to discuss the result of your biopsy. Neng, I am very sorry that I am the one that has to tell you this – the result is positive. You have squamous

carcinoma. You are probably scared and thinking that you are going to die, yes of course you have all the right to have those feelings, but Neng I will promise you that we will fight this disease. Inday Fe and me will make sure that you will get all the help you need. I got in touch with Dr. Palmares, and you can come to her clinic and I suggested if we could have a virtual meeting along with Jonelle and Toto Boy to discuss options and I will ask her to refer you to a good Oncologist so that we can start the treatment right away. Toto Boy, What I would ask for you is to be there for my sister. Be a sounding board of support for her. She needs you more than ever now - all of us to stand by her side," I explained with my heart breaking looking at my sister, how terrified she was.

"Inday Buday, I will leave to you and Inday Fe the fate of Miniang [the name my brother in-law fondly calls my sister], as we have no means to afford her treatment. We can't rely on Jonelle and Rochelle as they have difficulties making ends meet in England." My brother-in-law cried.

"Inday Fe and I will try everything humanly possible to give her the best care and for her to be comfortable. I am not there, so, what I am asking all of you, who are there by her side - especially you Toto Boy because you're her husband. Take care of her. She will be needing a lot of support from you." Speaking directly to my brother-in-law.

Then, I turned my attention to my sister who was crying, inconsolable. She was devastated upon hearing the bad news, who won't be?

"Neng, look at me please! Listen, I don't pretend that I know how you feel at this moment; you're sad,

131

angry and you might be thinking that you are going to die, you have all the right to express those feelings. Cry until you runout of tears, scream [forget you can talk], be angry until you run out of steam. But please I beg you, don't give up fighting. We will fight this evil disease until the end. I love you so much Neng and I will always be here for you. I will call you when you wake up in the morning and before you go to bed. Don't worry about anything. Let me know whatever you need, or anything else," Trying to be strong for her.

She scribbled again on the pad; took her a couple of minutes before she finished what she wanted to say. Lorna, her devoted caregiver, read it for her.

"Bud's thank you so much for helping me. I don't want to die yet if possible. I still want to see MC and UK graduates get married and have their own family. I am still too young to die," she said crying.

"Neng, You are my sister and I love you. I will do everything in my power to help you, but we have also to accept that there are things that are out of our control, and one of them is death. We have to pray that God will give you the courage to face whatever it is that He instilled for you. In the meantime, cherish and live your life, don't let the cancer rob you of the moment to be happy with your family, regardless of the circumstances. Hang on to your faith," Encouraging her.

"Ate Lori, Mama has an appointment to see her ENT [I can't put names without their permission] on Friday, June 4 @2PM. So, maybe if you could make an appointment for Mama to see Dr. Palmares, that would save Mama another trip to the city," Lorna suggested.

"Okay, I will try to see if she can take you on Friday at noon. I will let you know," replying to her suggestion.

I felt better after I talked to my sister, and in knowing that she knows everything and she can start the process of accepting and coping with having cancer. It was very difficult and emotionally draining, but I did it.

Meanwhile, I got another message from Dr. Palmares confirming that she received the biopsy report. She expressed empathy and was extremely helpful; answered all my questions patiently. Without wasting any time, she referred my sister to an oncologist.

"Thank you so much, Dr. Palmares for all your help and assistance – I will be forever grateful to you! Thank you for always being there for my family [she had been my youngest brother's doctor and medical advisor], she never hesitates to help my brother and my other siblings whenever a medical problem arises," expressing my gratitude.

"No problem, Ms. Pilatan. I hope Mrs. Maquiling will be okay. We will try to get her help, just encourage her to be positive and pray," sounding optimistic.

"I am trying to be optimistic under the circumstances. However, sometimes it's hard to be optimistic when you see your loved ones suffer. By the way, Doctor, my sister, has an appointment with her ENT on June 4, 2pm; can she come that day at 12 or after she finishes with her ENT so that she does not need to come back again?" I asked.

"My clinic opens at noon until 4pm. Ask Mrs. Maquiling to come before 12. I will try to speak to her

ENT, he is just 2 doors down from my clinic. Regarding the virtual meeting, I have no problem just that the connection sometimes is not great," she replied.

I was thankful, and extremely pleased with the result of our conversation. Somehow, I like Dr. Palmares, she is very easy to talk to; she is attentive – pays attention to your concern and promptly addresses it.

My sister was very ecstatic when I told her that I made an appointment for her to see Dr. Palmares at12, then followed by her ENT. I also let her know the good news that there is already a referral for her to see an Oncologist and hopefully she could start her treatment very soon. As I promised - I called her twice a day to check on her; in the morning when she woke up and in the evening before she went to bed. Sometimes, she was very depressed and hardly wrote anything on her pad [it's her way of communication], since the surgery. I would read her a scripture, or some positive and uplifting quotations – some from mine collections, and some are from well-known philosophers. Or I would read her a poem from my book "Poem collection: a reflection of my life". She would smile while I was reading it for her, then she would scribble what she wanted to say and would ask Lorna or Myra to read it to me. At the end of our conversation, she would blow me a kiss.

I left a message for Rochelle [my nephew's wife] about the virtual meeting which is going to take place at Dr. Palmares' clinic at noon, on June 4. She replied to me that they will try to be there, regardless of the difficulties because of the different time zones.

I did all my research and prepared all the questions I'd like to ask Dr. Palmares, although most of the questions had been answered by her, just a formality's sake and for my sister and Toto Boy's benefit. Unfortunately, the connections were very bad; it is difficult to hear what the other person is saying from the other line – a lot of static! So, I decided to end the conversation as I found it meaningless. I left a message for Dr. Palmares to just update me on what had been discussed during the course of their virtual meeting with my nephew, and my sister and brother-in-law.

The next morning, I received a message from my messenger from Dr. Palmares, updating me of their virtual meeting. According to her the meeting went well - Neneng Herminia will make an appointment with her oncologist and hopefully she will be able to start her treatment right away. She would also follow-up it with her. All Neneng's medical records have been sent to her as requested, including the biopsy. I called Lorna to remind her to make an appointment to the oncologist as soon as possible.

"Good evening, Lorna! How's everything there? Did you make an appointment with the oncologist?" I quired.

"Yes, Ate Lori. Mama had an appointment to see the oncologist next week, but we need to have an antigen covid-19 test within 48 hours prior to going there. They have very strict rules there Ate; only me can accompany Mama; Papa Boy is not allowed to come up with us," she explained in detail.

"Let me speak to your Mama Neng, please." She handed the phone to Neneng.

Good evening, Neng! You're looking nice. Have you eaten your dinner yet?" I asked.

Scribbled in a pad, for a couple of minutes or so then, handed the pad to Lorna to read for me.

"Yes, I had my dinner, but I can't eat much as my throat bothered me; it feels tight and when I drink fluid I coughed," she explained through Lorna.

"Well, we can remedy the tightness on your throat – lubrication [joking]. The coughing is the one that you have to watch out for because if it persists you may be you need to thicken your fluid intake a bit to prevent aspiration. You could have pneumonia if the fluid gets into your lung, but then you know that Neng right? You're a nurse, so you are well aware of those things." An open-ended question.

She scribbles in the pad again, writing her thoughts and other things that she would like to say to me. Watching her in this scene made me so sad – my poor sister, isn't she suffering enough? But I tried to be strong for her. I told all my cousins, nephews and nieces [in Canada and the Philippines] to video call her as for her to feel that she is not alone; her family are behind her in this journey. After she finished writing she handed the paper to Lorna for her to read.

"Thank you Bud's for always calling me and making me laugh even though it's very hard at times. I am very lucky to have you as my sister and I want you to know that I appreciate and am grateful for everything that you are doing for me. I know you are working hard there, just to support me and my needs." She was crying again as Lorna read what she had written down.

"Neng, I don't want you to think about money. You are more important to us [Inday Fe and me], God is good Neng; He always provides. He gives us trials,

136

but He always provides for us to get by and overcome our predicament. We just need to learn to accept our situation and trust His will in our lives. It's difficult to understand sometimes, but no matter what happens we must cling to His promises That "He will not give us trials beyond what we can handle, but if He did – He will provide a way for us to overcome it. And He will never, never abandon us, in our hours of need," trying to lift her spirit up.

She scribbled again in her pad, so intently for a few seconds then asked Lorna to read it for me.

"I tried to cling to my faith and believed that this is just a trial for me, but I have been through so much that it's hard sometimes to be optimistic," she uttered dejectedly.

"Take it one day at a time, Neng. We are here for you, to support and to love you. we are in this together. By the way, I sent you money for your weekly allowance. You have to try and eat healthy and nutritious food to prepare your body for your treatment. Maybe you should drink some Ensure to supplement what you're missing in your meal." I suggested.

"Yes, Ate Lori, that's what I am about to suggest. Mama needs to have some extra supplement to prepare her body for the treatment," Lorna added.

"I sent money this morning, the control number was in your messenger. Give it to your papa Boy, then buy her ensure and whatever she wants to eat and medical supplies. Encourage her to have more fruits and vegetables. Please, call me when you get to the oncologist office and tell the doctor that I want to speak

to her to discuss my sister's diagnosis and the plan of treatment," giving Lorna Instruction.

As usual, before the end of our conversation my sister forced a smile and blew me a kiss. I noticed that she was more at peace than the first few weeks. I just kept encouraging her to be hopeful; to take it one day at a time. In the meantime, she has to live her life and try to savor every moment of it. Most of all, to accept God's will whatever that might be. I encouraged her to read the scriptures, sometimes I read it with her.

The day my sister was going to see the oncologist, I was already prepared for all my questions. Because of different time zones, Wednesday 2 pm in the Philippines, it's Tuesday 2am in Canada, as Philippines is twelve hours ahead. I had waited and waited for a call from Lorna, and finally my cell rang at 2:49, almost three o'clock. Telling me that the doctor had no time to talk to me as she was extremely busy. I was pissed, I guess I am used to being here in Canada where doctors met with the family to explain the disease, how far it went, what it means, and the course or plan of treatment. Well of course, it is absurd for me to compare the two countries, as the Philippines is still considered a third world country, whereas Canada, although our healthcare system is not perfect but still considered as one of the best in the world. Lorna updated me with what the oncologist did, well absolutely nothing! She blurted out, "you have cancer!" I knew that, everybody knows that, [maybe I am exaggerating a bit; not everybody]. My poor sister had to travel 33 kilometers just to be told that she had cancer- which she knows already. What a joke!

What we were hoping to know from this doctor, is to tell us her plan on how to treat my sister, we do not even know what stage of cancer my sister had. But the thing that ticked me off is the rudeness of these doctors – the lack of compassion and empathy. I think some doctors in the Philippines don't practice the concept of holistic medicine well. That the whole person is made up of interdependent parts and if one is not working properly, all parts will be affected. Therefore, doctors should not only address the illness but as well as the emotional, psychological, spiritual and wellbeing of their patients with respect and dignity. I think one the root causes are Classism – if you have the money and connection [like a politician] in the Philippines you will be treated like royalty; however, if you are poor and downtrodden, you will end up in the gutter. I am not saying that all doctors in Canada are on their best behavior, of course we have few of those rude and arrogant doctors too. The only difference - in Canada we don't discriminate against people based on their status; everybody is treated equally. In Canada we value and respect the dignity of every person, regardless of their stature. So far the only doctor that earned my respect and admiration is Dr. Rosalinda Palmares.

I don't like being a pest, but I need to for my sister's sake. I am fighting for her life. I message Doctora Palmares, that I need her to find me a new oncologist because I don't like the one that she referred to my sister. Likewise, I am pushing for my sister to start her treatment as soon as possible.

"Lori, I could refer Mrs. Maquiling to St. Paul Hospital [Iloilo] Cancer Center. They have a complete facility there, including a Radiation machine, which we don't have here at Mission. She could have both

chemo and radiation there at the same time," she suggested.

"I would be forever indebted to you Doctor if you could help my sister to speed up for her to start her treatment, it would be great. I am worried that the longer she waits the more the cancer will get a chance to advance and spread. However, if my sister will do the treatment at St Paul, I still would like to retain you as my sister's attending physician," I reiterated.

"No problem, I am also affiliated at St. Paul Hospital," she replied.

"Thank you so much Doctor. Please find out for me the cost of this treatment so that I can prepare the money," asking her a favor.

"I will try to stop by the Cancer Center tomorrow after my rounds. Just give me until the end of the week and I will have all the answers for you," she stated.

I felt better after my conversation with Dr. Palmares. She is really awesome; always going out of her way to accommodate me, in spite of her busy schedules: she teaches at Doctors' College of Medicine, affiliated with a few hospitals in the city, and has a clinic at Mission Hospital and her hometown. She was truly an amazing woman; tireless and dedicated to her profession, not to mention compassionate and empathetic. Qualities and traits that the majority of Filipino doctors are missing. My sister was ecstatic when I shared her good news.

"Thank you, Bud's for tirelessly doing your best to help me." Lorna said, reading what had written in the pad.

"I told you Neng, that I will do my best to help you. We are all in this together as a family. Always remember that," reassuring her again.

At the end of the week Dr. Palmares, left a message in my messenger that she spoke to the head of cancer radiologist at Cancer Center at St. Paul Hospital, Doctor D. She forwarded him all the information and biopsy report he needs to know for him to decide what's the best treatment for my sister. She left his contact number for me to get in touch with him. After thanking Dr. Palmares, I sent a message to Doctor D introducing myself as Mrs. Maquiling sister, and would greatly appreciate it if he could get back to me in his own convenient time to discuss my sister's cancer and most of all how to proceed from here on – her treatment.

I was surprised how quickly he got back at me. I asked permission if I can call him on his messenger? He replied back that I may.

"Hi Doctor D! My name is Lori Pilatan, I am Mrs. Maquiling's sister. Thank you so much for getting back to me so quickly. I guessed, at the stage of the game, you already know what you're up against. I am sure Dr. Palmares has briefed you about my sisters and sent you all the reports and diagnosis of her cancer," I said bluntly.

"Yes, ma'am Lori. As a matter of fact, we had discussed what would be the best possible course of treatment – most likely – the combination of Radiation and chemotherapy. However, prior to her receiving treatment we need to prepare the body, which means we need to ensure that the body is strong enough to withstand the treatment," he explained thoroughly.

"First of all, please don't call me ma'am, it makes me sound old. Lol! In a serious note, any suggestion you have, you can run it by with Dr. Palmares because I give her full authority to speak on our behalf. Likewise, you have my full support whatever it is you think that will give my sister a chance for life." I stated my full support.

"I think before Mrs. Maquiling will start the treatment we have to put her on a feeding tube - to ensure that her body will receive enough nutrients to fight the side effects of chemo and radiation." He explained.

"I am well aware of different kinds of feeding tubes - if it's not going to be an issue of her receiving nutrients on her body, I would prefer for her to have a PEG, instead of Nasogastric [NG] tube for quality-of-life purposes. The other question I want to raise is, can it be reversed once the treatment is over and she gets better?" asking him straight forward.

"Yes it can be reversed, I don't see why not once she started eating on her own and hopefully survives her cancer. But you have to talk to Doctora Palmares about it and discuss it with her," he replied.

"Doctor, will you please tell me how much it will cost for both the treatment - chemo and radiation?" I queried.

"I will ask the clerk to prepare a costing summary for Mrs. Maquiling's treatment. As well as, I will discuss this further to Dr. Palmares and Doctor A, [your sister's new oncologist]. You can message him through his messenger fb account," he patiently responded

After thanking him for his insight and answering my questions, I left Dr. Palmares a message on her messenger regarding my discussion with Doctor D, about my sister having a feeding tube and about Doctor A, if she knew him. After half an hour, I received a message from her that she is at school right now [she teaches at Doctor Hospital, College of medicine], but she will call me back as soon as she gets home. Doctor Palmares is always good at her promises; kept her words. An hour later she called me through messenger.

"Good evening Lori. Yes, we discussed the feeding procedure for Mrs. Maquiling prior to her undergoing treatment to ensure that her body gets proper nutrition to withstand the side effects of chemo and radiation. We also talked about her need to have her dental check as to prevent oral complications. And I had spoken to Doctor A, and he sounded very nice and insightful. I also talked to Doctor V, gastroenterologist [specializing in digestive system]. We are just waiting for a go-ahead signal from you; when do you want it done?" she explained thoroughly.

"Well, the earlier the better, isn't it Doctor?" I replied.

"Of course, absolutely! Ask Mrs. Maquiling's caregiver to make an appointment to see Doctor V, as he wants to see her before the procedure," she further added.

After my conversation with Dr. Palmares I called my sister to let her know of the newest development. She looked very excited while I was talking. I also asked Lorna to make an appointment with the gastroenterologist as he wants to see her prior to performing the procedure. The doctor saw Neneng, and he booked the PEG insertion on June 7, 2021. I requested for Doctora Palmares to put her in a private room. I don't know what I would have done without the help of this kind hearted doctor. She facilitated everything and walked me through it, explained everything patiently and made sure I understood everything.

My sister had her PEG insertion procedure done, and everything went so well that she was discharged from the hospital 3 days later to recuperate at home. Thank God, we are blessed with a caring and very knowledgeable caregiver in the person of Lorna. The first week my sister had difficulties adjusting to the new changes; not able to taste her food. PEG allows nutrition, fluids and/ or medication to be put directly into the stomach, bypassing the mouth and esophagus. She missed those feelings of tasting and chewing her food. When she told me this, it made me extremely sad; I felt so sorry for her. but I had to hide my feelings as I couldn't afford to fall apart. The other thing that she was complaining about was that she couldn't sleep, as she needs to be fed every 4 hours. I called Dr. Palmares if the feeding time could be adjusted so that she doesn't need to be awake when she is already sleeping.

"We can do that; I don't see why," she replied.

Dr. Palmares changed the feeding schedule of my sister to allow her to sleep undisturbed during the night. She was looking much better, in fact, if you just looked at her you're not going to suspect that she has cancer. She is more relaxed and I think she started to accept the fact that she had cancer and learn to cope with it as she battles to survive the disease. Calling her twice a day made it also easier for her in knowing that she is not alone in this battle; her family were standing by her side.

Things were starting to move in the right direction: she had her PEG procedure done, her teeth were all checked; cleaned and put filling in, and her dentist put dentures on her missing front teeth. In the meantime, I received the costing summary from St. Paul Iloilo Cancer Center, detailing how much it was going to cost for my sister's treatment, not including the chemotherapy which will be done by her oncologist [doctor A]. I was told that The Cancer Center policy is "you pay as you go" – you pay after each treatment. They're ready to start the treatment anytime. They're just waiting for my go-ahead signal [financially]. I told them that the money had been sent to my sister. Doctor D and Doctor A had sent me a message on my messenger that the three of them discussed [Dr. Palmares, Doctor A and Doctor D] to start my sister's chemo treatment on July 28,2021, followed by Radiation on July 29, 2021. She will be receiving radiation Monday-Friday. Weekend breaks to allow normal cells to recover, and chemo once a week for four months. I was so ecstatic to hear the good news – finally Neneng Herminia will start her treatment. I was so excited to tell her this encouraging news.

"Good morning Neng, you are looking great. Can you smile with your new teeth?" teasing her.

"Good morning Bud's! Thank you for everything." She smiles back as Lorna reads what she had written in the pad.

"By the way, I have some good news to tell you; I spoke to Doctor A and Doctor D and they arranged *for you to start your chemo on July 28, followed by radiation. Your chemo is only [X1] in a week, while your radiation is going to be Monday to Friday for four months,"* I explained

She scribbled down on a pad for a few minutes, then handed it to Lorna for her to read to me.

"Bud's, will chemo drugs cause my hair to fall out?" she asked worriedly.

"Not all, however, most chemo patients lose their hair after 2 to 3 weeks of starting treatment. But don't worry about it, it's just a hair. It will grow back up again," reassuring her.

"I hope I am going to respond to treatment and get better because I don't want to die yet Bud's." She was crying while Lorna was reading what she had written in the pad.

"Neng, we have to believe that you would. But whatever happened we are here for you. It's okay to be scared of death, however you should know that every human being dies. Death is coming whether we like it or not - it is inevitable. It's just a question of when and how, like what happened to our siblings; the four of them died so young and the nature of their death was horrible that it took me a while to accept it. I believe that each one of us has our own timetable; when our life expires. So, instead of fearing death, we should find our purpose and meaning and enjoy life to the fullest. Don't waste your time every waking hour thinking, "I am going to die" rather, make it meaningful by doing things that you would like to do, or spend quality time with your loved ones. We are going to support you whatever

it is that you would like to do," reassuring her but telling her as it is.

To support and maybe amuse her, the next day I went to the parlor and had my hair shaved off. Then, call her in the evening, as I always do; call her twice a day- when she wakes up in the morning and before she goes to bed. She burst laughing when she saw my bald head.

"What have you done to your hair? You look like you're about to sit in the electric chair." She was laughing while Lorna was reading what she had written on her communication pad.

"I told you; I am with you on this journey. So, just in case you lost your hair, you have company - me!" laughing out loud!

She started her treatment; a combination of chemo and radiation. Things started well for the first two months. She has no side effect symptoms; unfortunately, she was positive for covid, even though she had covid vaccine. We were so worried for her because she is very fragile and vulnerable. Thank God the symptoms were very mild. The treatment resumed on September 20, 2021 after her fourteen-day quarantine. However, there was another setback – the radiation machine broke and needs to be sent to Manila to have it fixed, which means another delay in her treatment – three weeks. Finally, in spite of ebb and flow she completed her treatment on October 14, 2021. All the laboratories are looking in the right direction; a lot of improvement. Doctor Palmares, Doctor A and doctor D could never be pleased with the encouraging result. We were told to wait for three months for her to have a scan to make sure that she was truly responding to treatment.

Neneng Herminia is extremely happy and feeling good. There is a glimmer of hope, that things will get better and she will survive this horrible disease. To help her boast her self-image I asked Lorna to arrange for someone to come to the house to have her hair, nails and foot done. "sickness is an affront to one's self-image and dignity". You look better, you feel better. I was teasing her when I called.

"Wow, Neng, I hardly didn't recognize you. The majority of cancer patient's looked horrible, you on the other hand are blooming." I was clowning around but *she really looks good.*

"That's because of your generosity and kindness. I am so lucky to have a sister like you. Thank you for actively participating in my treatment even though you are there in Canada," she said almost in tears.

"Neng, don't forget Inday Fe, she helped out too," reminding her.

My sister tried her best to have a sense of normalcy, regardless of her physical condition. It must be hard not to be able to talk; the only way to communicate is to scribble in a pad to express what you wanted to say. And the feeding tube makes it even worse. When I called her I could sense the frustration written all over her face but she would try to hide it, not to disappoint me. However, she did better than the previous months. I encourage her to read, go out so that she can get at least some fresh air.

"Neng, why don't you go to the beach - not that far from where you live. You have a car; it makes it easier for you to travel," encouraging her.

148

"Bud's I tried not to spend the money unwisely, for I know how hard you were working for it. I feel bad that you have to spend all your hard-earned money for me, if only I had the means, unfortunately, I don't have the capacity financially and neither does Jonelle. Everything is very expensive here, especially the gas." She looks dejected while Lorna was reading what she had written

"Don't worry about me Neng, and I don't want you to feel guilty about it. If the table were reversed, wouldn't you try anything to help me? How about I will give you an extra five thousand for your outing?" I stated.

"Thank you Bud's!" She was teary while Lorna read it.

It's not easy financially, as she needs three kinds of formula on her feeds [ensure gold, anlene gold and another one], each cost about over two-thousand pesos; that's six thousand pesos for three. She needs [x2] each of those in a week which means for the feeds alone it cost about twelve thousand pesos, added to that were her medical supplies, doctors, laboratories, and covid test [as it was the height of covid during that time]. Her twenty thousand allowances for a week [not including the caregiver salary] is barely enough to meet all her needs. Added to that is scan and other imaging required. Inday Fe helped out and Jonelle and his wife volunteered to pay the caregiver's salary. But one thing I learned throughout my journey, that God is a good provider. A lot of things we don't understand, but at the end of the day, God is true to all his promises; we are never left without help. On January 4,2022, Neneng had her laboratories and CT scan. The result was very encouraging. The cancer shrunk and the laboratory result was normal. Doctor A and Doctor Palmares even suggested that she should practice eating bit by bit and swallowing because she is going to have another CT scan in June and if everything goes well they will remove the feeding tube. My sister was in seventh heaven upon hearing it. She was so excited; her eyes lit up when we were talking about it. Everything seemed to be working well, then Lorna messaged me that she is only up until the end of January as they were going to move to the city. She had a heavy heart leaving my sister, but she had no choice as her husband works during the day and she has to stay home to take care of her toddler child. The news was not received by my sister well, as she had grown to love Lorna. She was very good to her – treated her like her mother. With Lorna, she did not have to worry as she is very conscientious and knowledgeable: cleaning trach, cleaning and flushing her feeding tube, taking vital signs, putting oxygen and making appointments for my sister, but most and foremost she addressed the emotional needs of my sister by talking to her and she treated her with respect and dignity.

I have to post on one of those caregiver sites, and interview dozens of people from here, but none were even half as good as Lorna. I was so frustrated and exasperated. Anyway, since Lorna left, my sister had five different caregivers – some lasted only a week, others just a few days. My nephew Ryan and his girlfriend have to pitch in to take care of her sometimes. Every time I called she had a barrage of complaints, and criticisms about her caregiver; whether they were lazy, sloppy, brainless or a thief, and etc.

"Wow, Neng, it seems like you have all kinds of characters, maybe we could make a movie out of them. What role would you like to be, a villain or a victim?" laughing out loud!

She would smile, but I could sense her frustration, but what was worrisome when I paid attention to her face, she had this pensive sad look on her face.

"Neng, are you okay? Is there anything you're not telling me?" I asked worriedly.

She scribbled on her communication pad for about a couple of minutes, then handed it to Myra [our great niece], to read.

"I have some pain in my back. Sometimes, I am awakened during the night. It hurts when I cough. Then my throat seemed very tight," she said in a melancholic tone.

"Since when?" I queried.

"About two weeks ago. The symptoms are gradually increasing," said Myra reading what she had written.

"You should have told me any symptoms you had right away. Anyway, I will book an appointment for you to see Doctora Palmares. About these caregivers, don't worry I will address it, I will make sure that they will do what they've been hired to do," reassuring her.

After I finished my conversation with her, I messaged Doctora Palmares and her oncologist about this new development - this was sometimes in May. I booked an appointment for her to see both her oncologist and

Doctor Palmares. In the meantime, I encouraged her to sit up and walk around as much as possible to prevent pneumonia. Doctor Palmares, messaged me that she saw Neneng Herminia and she prescribed her with an antibiotic and cough syrup for her cough. Her oncologist requested for her to have an earlier CT scan after he saw her.

I was on a tenterhook awaiting the CT scan result, as every time I talked to her I could see changes in her facial expression and I didn't like the sound of her cough. Likewise, she complained about tightness on her trach and she said it's very painful at times. She hardly gets any sleep at night. I had very bad feelings about this – something bad is about to happen.

After two weeks my nephew and his girlfriend picked up the CT scan result at St. Paul. I gave them the instruction to send it to me right away. Reading the result, I couldn't help but shed a tear- feeling sorry for my sister. She was hopeful that things will work out; in fact, she was excited that after this CT scan she will start to eat again – no more feeding tube. Instead, the cancer has metastasized through her lungs and it's grown bigger than it was. How am I going to find the strength and courage to tell my sister – that her cancer came back with a vengeance, this time it metastasis on her lung. On the other hand; I have no choice but to tell her the truth.

"Good evening Neng! How are you feeling today?" I asked nervously.

"I didn't sleep last night; I was coughing and my back hurts and I was congested from the phlegm. Ryan told me that you had the result of the CT scan, what is it?" she queried.

"Neng, I am so sorry but the cancer came back, and this time it is worse than what it was; it has spread through your lungs. That's the reason that your back hurts and you were coughing a lot. And the mass on your throat grew bigger, that's why you were feeling the tightness there. I am so sorry, that I am the bearer of bad news to you. I know you are extremely disappointed because this is not the outcome that we are hoping for," I said somberly.

She was so quiet, no emotion or anything. She just sat there dejectedly.

"Neng, please talk to me, say something. We are not giving up. We are still going to fight this wherever it's going to take us," trying to encourage her to cling to hope.

She thought for a moment, then scribbles on her communication pad for a couple of minutes or more. When she finished she handed it to Lorna to read for me. [She came back to work for Neneng Herminia, as she felt sorry for what she had to go through with different caregivers].

"Thank you Bud's. But I made up my mind that I am not going to seek further treatment anymore. I have to accept that soon I am going to die. Instead of wasting your hard-earned money for my treatment I would like to ask you if you don't mind continuing to continue providing my weekly allowance for my feeds and my other medical needs. When I get a bit stronger I would like to go home to the farm, then visit Nene Ditay [our eldest sibling who lives farther away, part of Dumarao]," She said, determined.

"Neng, is that what you really want? I will support whatever decision you decide," trying to compose myself and be strong for her.

"Yes, Bud! I already made up my mind. I already accepted my fate and surrendered my life to God. I'd like to use whatever time I have to spend some quality time with my family and savor every moment of it," she clearly stated. Crying while Lorna was reading what she had written.

"Very well, Neng. I will convey your wishes to Doctor Palmares and to your oncologist," I said sadly.

After I finished my conversation with my sister, I messaged Doctora Palmares and her oncologist that we will not seek further treatment anymore. My sister had already made up her mind. Doctora Palmares, tried to explain to me that if she does not seek treatment, the cancer might advance rapidly and spread out in other parts of her body and she will suffer even more. Especially the one on her throat – it could grow bigger and block the larynx completely. Same opinion expressed by her oncologist. He suggested chemo pills as opposed to intravenous infusions. It's more convenient; she does not need to go to the hospital for it. She just takes the chemo pills as prescribed.

"I appreciated all the efforts, but I can't decide for my sister. I cannot force her to do things that she is not comfortable doing. After all, it is her life that we are talking about. The only thing that I can do is to relay both your concerns to her," I replied to them both.

Thinking about the two doctors' opinions and suggestions makes sense. The last thing I want to see is for her to suffer. At least with the chemo pills, it would probably help stabilize her cancer, preventing it from getting worse. I made up my mind to tell her what Doctora Palmares and doctor A had said. The next morning when I called her, as I always do every day.

"Good morning Neng! I had spoken to Doctora Palmares and Doctor A, I told them that you're not going to seek treatment. And they both explained; that if you are not going to seek further treatment the cancer might spread like a wildfire spreading all over your body and would cause more suffering for you. They both suggested for you to have chemo pills; which means that you don't have to go to the hospital because it is just like an ordinary pill – you take it as prescribed. No more poking of needles. It's more of a comfort measure, and who knows if miracles do happen. But I leave it up to you to decide, Neng. Whatever decision you have, I will support it," telling it as it was explained to me.

She scribbled on her writing pad, or communication pad for about two minutes, then she handed it to Myra for her to read to me.

"Bud's, what is the use of taking those chemo pills if I am not going to get better? I will cling to a false hope that maybe I will get better, but I am not! Besides, I pity you already for working hard just to pay for my treatment and medical expenses – you and Inday Fe," crying while Myra was reading what she had written.

"Neng, don't worry about money, you are more important. Inday Fe and I will earn it again if we are healthy. The most important thing is that you are comfortable and don't suffer. If you ask me, I would agree with Doctor Palmares and Doctor A. But then

again, it's your life, it's your decision, Neng." I reiterated that money is not an issue.

"Okay, Bud's if that's what you think and the doctors are best for me, I would go for it. So, when can I start taking the chemo pills?" She smiled at me while Myra read what she had written.

"I will message Doctora Palmares and Doctor A, then I will see, but I assume soon," I replied.

I messaged both Doctor Palmares and Doctor A, telling them that my sister had finally agreed to take the chemo pills. Doctor A and I had a conversation through messenger that he is going to order the chemo pills. In the meantime, while we are waiting for the pills we can buy it from the pharmacy, but before she starts taking it, he'd like to see her in his clinic to make sure that everything's good. My sister will receive 6 sessions. Fourteen [14] days of taking the pills consistently, then seven days rest – that's one session, until she finishes the whole 6 sessions.

Lorna accompanied my sister to see Dr. A – vital signs were okay. He gave her requisition for Laboratory to check her liver function, her red blood cell [RBC], white blood cell [WBC] and platelet counts before she could have to start taking the chemo pills. If everything went well, she could start the treatment right away.

She started taking her chemo pills [Xeloda] 500mg tablets, on July 12,2022 and she completed one session on July 26, 2022. She seemed to have tolerated it – no side effects. She was becoming hopeful again because she started feeling better; the tightness on her larynx or throat seemed to have decreased and so was the coughing and the pain in her back. After she had rested for seven days, she started on her second session on August 3,2022. However, after one week on her second session she had experienced side effects [LBM], and she looked lethargic and weak every time I video called her through messenger.

"Neng, are you okay?" I was concerned.

"My stomach is bloated all the time and tired of going back and forth to the washroom. And my cough seems to have come back - I can't sleep at night because of it." She looked sad while Lorna was reading what she had written.

"How about your throat? Would you like me to make an appointment for you to see Doctor A and Doctor Palmares?" I asked.

"Ate, maybe after Mama finishes her second session for which she is due next week, August 16. She has a laboratory schedule on August 18. Then, I will book an appointment for her to see Doctor A before she starts her third session," Lorna suggested.

"That makes sense, what do you think, Neng?" I asked, looking at her which she nodded in agreement.

My sister was determined to finish the treatment that she endured the side effects of it [LBM], and among other things. She did finish the second session on August 16,2022. After her laboratory – she was a bit on the low side, however, Doctor A, thinks that she is okay to proceed for her third [3] session. Seven days break will help her to recuperate from the chemo drugs before she starts on the next session. I was troubled by what I was seeing, but I tried to keep it to myself. I don't think that she is responding to the treatment, even my sister in-law expressed sadness every time they went to see her. At some point, my niece had to run outside to cry when my sister had an episode of paroxysmal coughing which caused her to struggle to breathe.

I expressed this concern to both Doctor A and Doctora Palmares, in which they both tried their best to address the issues, but look doctors are not God; they have limitations in which they can do. Doctora Palmares referred her to a palliative doctor for pain management and likewise to help her cope with the possibility of death – "end of life". I knew in my heart that we are losing this battle. It's excruciating to watch her suffer. I love my sister with all my heart and God knows Inday Fe and I tried our best to help her prolong her life, however I didn't like to see her in pain and suffering anymore. Whenever bad things happened to my family the first thing I asked God "why?", but this time I didn't question His power anymore, I just prayed that He would spare my sister from further suffering. She had been through so much the last few years of her life which deprived her of quality of life. First, her leg surgery, then the car accident which took away her mobility. And the final stroke is the cancer which took away her voice to speak [can you imagine for someone who like to talk and lost your voice, must be devastating] and not be able to taste the food to satisfied your craving because you have to be tube feeding or "enteral nutrition" directly to your stomach or small intestine. Come to think of it, my sister is not really living, but just existing!

She was almost a week through her third session of her chemo pills, as I always routinely do. I called her twice a day – in the morning and in the evening. That particular Sunday evening, around seven O'clock – Toronto time. Sonya [my weekend client] and I just finished our dinner when she asked me, If I am going to call my sister as she wants to speak to her as well before she goes to bed. She had grown to like my sister, as she spoke to her every weekend when I am at work with her. Sonya was the most optimistic person I knew. She was a holocaust survivor, suffered from a number of surgeries, heart problems, Arthritis - a lot of aches and pains, but she never gave up; she was always optimistic and always tried her best to help herself even if it's difficult sometimes. She always tells my sister to cling to hope.

"Always pray, and don't give up dear because as long as you are alive, there is always hope. I always include you in my prayers," she would encourage my sister to be positive.

Neneng Herminia, thanked Sonya for her concerns and words of wisdom. Their conversation was interrupted as Sonya had to use the toilet. After I put her to sit in the john, I went back to talk to my sister. I noticed she looked so weak.

"Neng, what's wrong, are you in some kind of pain?" I queried.

She nodded, then she scribbled on her communication pad and handed it to our great niece to read, as Lorna hadn't come yet from her weekend off.

"I didn't sleep last night, from coughing and diarrhea since four o'clock this morning – I was in and out of the washroom," she complained.

"Diarrhea is one of the side effects of Xeloda. You have to drink liquid Neng, to replenish the fluid that you lost. The last thing you need is for you to be dehydrated as it could cause more problems. Let me speak to Toto Boy," I said concerned, alarmed of what I saw in her – she was very lethargic, pale and frail.

"Good morning, Bud's! I am worried about Miniang [his pet name for her]. she was been in and out of the washroom since four o'clock this morning," he expressed concern.

"Toto Boy, you have to go out and buy her Gatorade and Imodium. Wait, Sonya was calling me, I have to help her get ready for bed; once she is in bed I will call you back," Rushing to attend Sonya.

After I put Sonya to bed, I said goodnight to her and called my sister back. My brother In-law answered the phone.

"Hello, Buds, Miniang fell on the floor, as she was trying to stand up from the toilet. I had to pick her up and carry her back to bed. I told her to not attempt to go to the toilet anymore as she is very weak, but she doesn't want to listen." My brother-in-law expressed concerns.

"Neng, Toto boy was right. Don't worry about making it in bed. You are wearing a diaper, it's better for you to do it in bed rather than risk yourself getting hurt. Neng, if you are tired already, please tell me and I will talk to Doctor A and Doctor Palmares to stop the chemo. I don't want to see you like this. Just tell me and I will do it. I love you so much, Neng!" I said in tears.

160

She scribbled on her communication pad for a couple of minutes then handed it to our great niece to read.

"Day, I want to finish this session because I am still hoping for a miracle from God, but just in case I will not make it, I would like to thank you and Inday Fe for all the sacrifices that the two of you have made for me. I am immensely grateful from the bottom of my heart. Please, lookout for my family, especially the UK. Likewise, you have to make sure that Myra and Maricel stay here and finish their school. Bud's, please find it in your heart to forgive Jonelle [her son] because when I am gone you and Inday Fe would be a second mother to him." She was crying while Roselyn [our great niece] read what she had written.

"I promised, I will try to do what you've asked of me. For now, stop talking Neng, you have to save your energy. Would you like me to pray with you just, silently follow me," she nodded in agreement.

At this time, Lorna walked in as my brother-in-law was about to leave to buy her Gatorade and Imodium. Then Lorna stopped him.

"Pa, if you are going to the pharmacy, buy an extra oxygen tube as the one Mama Neng has, it's already dirty. It really needs replacement." She further gives Toto Boy an instruction.

In the meantime, I called Doctor Palmares through messenger about my sister's condition, and requested if she could prepare a private room for her as I wanted her to go to the hospital to be given an Intravenous fluid because I suspected that she had been dehydrated. She called me back saying that there is no private room available because Iloilo City has an outbreak of "acute gastroenteritis' and cholera. Most of the private rooms are occupied. If I want they can put her in the Emergency Room [ER].

"*Whatever is available, Doctora, as long as my sister will get admitted,*" I replied.

After I finished with my conversation with Doctor Palmares, I called Lorna back through Video call and I can see that she is really struggling to breathe. I asked Lorna to take her vital and oxygen level. Everything was on the low side: BP 56/50 mmHg, oxygen was 62%. And this time she was already unconscious. I called Doctor Palmares again to inform her that things were not looking good. Even if they were to try to take her to Iloilo, I don't think she would make it there - she suggested taking her to a local hospital in Barotac because right now what she needs is fluid. She told me she has a friend that works there – she gave me the name of her friend. She hung up the phone and promised to call me back once she spoke to her doctor friend. Less than a couple of minutes she calls me back.

'" *Lori, I spoke to my friend and I already gave her a heads up about Mrs. Maquiling. She is waiting for her there. Tell your brother-in-law and the caregiver to take your sister now and ask for the doctor as soon as they get to the hospital,*" Doctor Palmares instructed.

As I hung up the phone, Lorna called me to say that Neneng Herminia was not doing well, her oxygen level dropped and so had her Vital signs. I told her to take her to Barotac Nuevo Hospital ASAP. I gave her an instruction and the name of the doctor and to call me as soon as they get there as I want to talk to the doctor.

But before they left I asked Lorna to put the phone in Neneng Herminia's ear.

"Neng I don't know if you can hear me, but I just want you to know that we love you so much. If you are tired now, it's okay to go and rest. I love you!" My heart was broken, because I knew that probably would be my last word for her.

I was anxious, but accepted whatever lies ahead. My gut feelings tell me that is not going to be pleasant news. I closed my eyes and prayed for my sister and for her family.

"Lord, into thy loving hands, I commit my sister's life. Hold her hands, comfort her and give her peace to let go and surrender everything to you. If there is anything that she hasn't asked for forgiveness yet, I beg you to please forgive her. I love her, but I know you love her more than I do. Please take care of her and help all of us to accept whatever is your will for her. In Jesus name I pray, Amen!" I barely finished my prayer when my phone rang. It was Lorna.

"Ate Lori, Mama Neng is gone. She was already flatline when we got to the hospital. Papa Boy was telling the doctor and nurses to resuscitate her. No matter how I explained that Mama was dead he just ignored me. He was just crying Ate Lori," Lorna relayed in tears.

"Lorna, please give the phone to him," I requested.

"Bud's Miniang was dead! She left us already," He said crying.

"Toto Boy, I am very sorry. I wished that the outcome would be different, but we did try our best to help her and prolong her life. But there are things that are out of our control, and one of them is death. It's heartbreaking to think that we will not be able to see her again, but we have to accept it. We have to let her go and let her be," Trying to comfort my brother in-law, who was devastated by the loss of his wife - my sister.

After I spoke to my brother in-law I spoke to the doctor and nurses as they tried to revive my sister. I saw her body lift up as they applied the Automated External Defibrillator [AED] to her chest.

"Please, stop! My sister is dead! Please let her be. I want her to die with dignity." I was furious at them.

Looking at my sister, lying in the gurney I couldn't help but cry, however I am grateful to God that He granted my prayer request – my sister's death was swift. She did not suffer.

I messaged both Doctor Palmares and Doctor A that my sister had just expired. I thanked them both for their help and assistance during those difficult journeys of my sister's living with cancer. Especially Doctor Palmares, who has been a pillar of support throughout. She was always accommodating and extremely helpful. Went above and beyond the call of duty to help my sister and me cope with it. It was a difficult journey for my sister and the entire family; however, having Doctor Palmares as my sister's internist, her oncologist, doctor A and her oncologist/radiologist Doctor D made it a bit easier to navigate. The compassion and empathy they'd shown to my sister was extraordinary.

Neneng Herminia fought with valor until the end. She lived one year and two months after she was diagnosed with Squamous cell carcinoma of the Larynx or vocal cords. Cancer takes away her voice, but she found a way to communicate – through her communication pad. Took away her joy to savor her food, yet eventually, she learned to have accepted it. It was not easy in the beginning, but as she journeyed living with cancer she learned to live with it.

Wherever she is now, I am sure she is smiling, *"free at last!"*

Len [described in chapter 9]

A retired teacher, who was diagnosed of Gastro-intestinal Stroma Tumor [GIST]. A cancer "alivers", who turns his cancer experienced into a positive experienced; his cancer paved the way for him to reached his dreamt to go to Hawaii and enjoyed the paradise Island for two weeks.

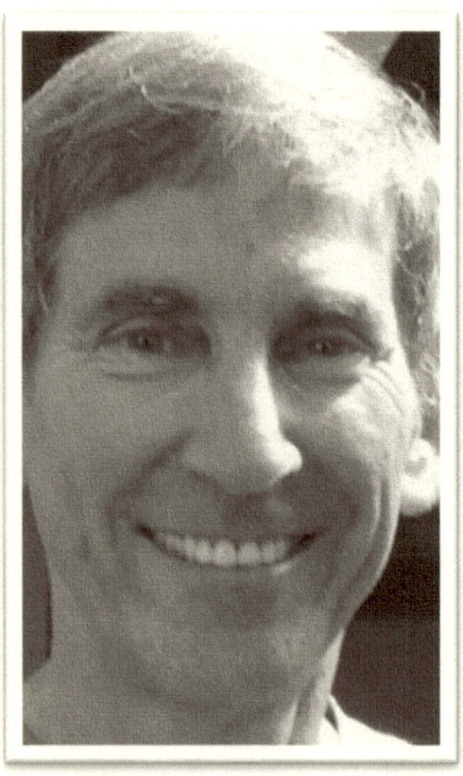

Chapter 9

Turning Lemon to Lemonade

This is a story of a friend of mine of his experience with getting cancer. Most of his life he had been healthy. He rarely got sick, and had not faced any major illnesses.

This situation changed when he was 62. He got flu-like symptoms, and he was having difficulty swallowing food when he ate. He went to see his GP [general practitioner] and was ordered to do some blood work to find out what's going on. His GP was concerned when his blood work came back and it showed an alarming drop of his hemoglobin level. He recommended that he have a gastroscopy done. He wasn't that concerned or expecting any surprises – he thought maybe it was just an ulcer that was causing the problems. When he went to get the gastroscopy he was sedated enough so that he wasn't aware of what was happening. When he started to awake from the sedation he was given some juice and a cookie while he was supposed to rest a bit before heading home.

The doctor who performed the gastroscopy came over to talk to him, it was about 4 o'clock in the afternoon, and apparently he was in a hurry to leave because even though he had bad news to deliver to him, he did not stay to answer any questions or offer any sympathetic advice or at least explain to him what he found out during the gastroscopy. Basically, the doctor said that he had a type of tumor, called GIST [gastro-intestinal stromal tumor], and there were two types it could be. One was very aggressive and dangerous, and he would die fairly quickly from it, but the other form was not as serious, and hopefully that's what he had. He told him to immediately arrange for a procedure to be done, as there were special centers in just a few hospitals in GTA or [Greater Toronto Area] that were performing this type of surgery. After he announced that, he left without even looking at him. He didn't stay even long enough to ask if he had any questions. This doctor behaves like he didn't care at all, for him he delivers the "bad news" and that's what it is? It's not his problem! What an idiot! No apathy or feeling. My friend was shocked, and scared. He was dismayed to learn that his problem was more serious than what he thought it was. He was terrified, thinking that he could be dead very soon.

Fortunately, has it turned out that the type of GIST he had was the lesser of two evils, however, the location of the tumor on his stomach, right beside the esophagus, meant that it would be complicated to remove the tumor because they had to cut part of the esophagus too. It meant severing the esophagus from the stomach, and then reattaching it. The removal of the sphincter between the stomach and esophagus meant that acid from the stomach would be an ongoing problem with reflux for the rest of his life.

The surgery went well, and then his worries turned to fear that the tumor might return. There was only one drug that was recommended to take, which would lessen the chance of tumor recurring [the drug called Gleevec], and he reluctantly agreed to take it. Every month, for the first year he had to return to the hospital for a CTScan, and to give blood samples. Needless to say, those appointments were very nerve-racking for him as he was fearing that they would find something. He was aware of how upset his stomach would be when he went to the appointment, and that he had no appetite, but as soon as he got the results of CTScan and blood test he got hungry, all of a sudden. So, the first year was extremely stressful, but the tumor had not returned and the blood tests showed everything was great except his hemoglobin levels. After the first year He had to return for tests every 3 months instead of monthly. Surviving the first year was a boost for his mood, but he really did not feel hopeful until 3 years had passed, and the surgeon who operated on him said that he is starting to feel hopeful about my friend surviving his cancer.

It wasn't until 5th year of having good results [he is still alive] that he truly started feeling relaxed about his situation and feeling that the worst was finally over. The oncologist, though, who was seeing him, was a depressive force for him, as she said the tumor was in remission, while he was hoping she would say that he likely wouldn't get cancer again. He was getting nervous with all the CT Scans he had been getting for the last five years, when she saw a small speck on his lung, in what was supposed to be his final CTScan, she recommended to monitor it. He only went back one time, and the speck had not changed, and she assured him it was not cancer. However, she wanted him to keep getting CTScans which my friend found ridiculous. So, he decided that he was done with the CTScan and with them, "tata, pip - pip, ciao!" He was more worried that the CTScans themselves were going to give him cancer.

One interesting result from all the expensive Gleevec he had been taking, was that he used his credit card to pay for it, but was getting reimbursed by his private insurance at work [he was a retired teacher, and their group insurance is one of the best in the country]. By the end of three years of getting Gleevec he had earned enough points to fly to the moon [just kidding], to Hawaii, or actually anywhere else in the world. However, it had always been his dream to go to Hawaii, and now that he felt he had recovered from his ordeal from cancer, and he had the free flight courtesy of Gleevec, he finally achieved his dream of going to Hawaii. My friend felt it was like the expression of "turning lemon into lemonade". His having cancer paved the way for the fulfillment of his dream to go to Hawaii.

On a serious note, my friend wished he had never gotten that cancer, and the problems with eating that he will be dealing with the rest of his life, but it sure was in seventh heaven to be in Hawaii for a couple of weeks.

Monina [describe in chapter 10]

A retired nurse, diagnosed of breast cancer. It's been over a year since she finished her last treatments. She was hoping that she would become one of those cancer "alivers", who could say, "I AM CANCER FREE!"

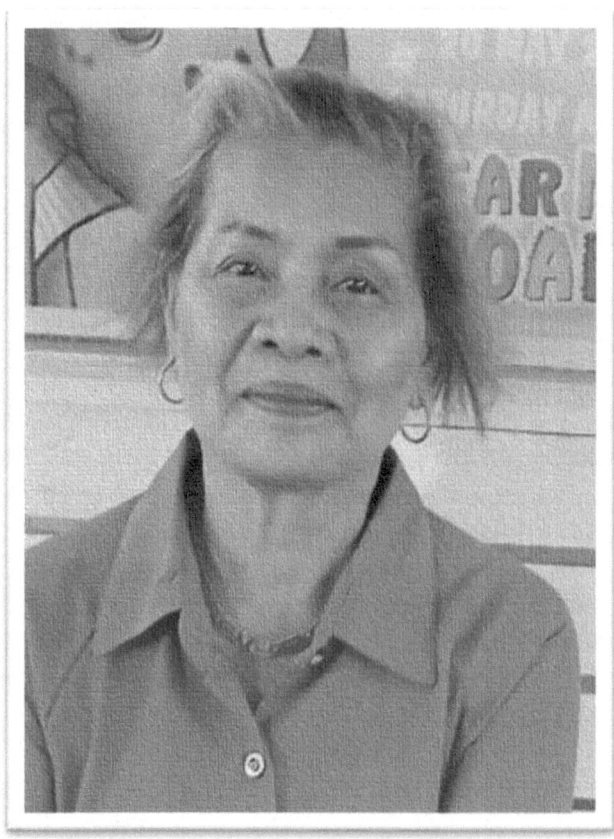

Chapter 10

Navigating through the storm

This is a story of my cousin, Monina Pascual Estandarte who was a retired Nurse at King Abdul Aziz University Hospital, Riyadh, Saudi Arabia. She worked there from September, 1980 and retired in 2012. She started as a staff nurse, then promoted to become a head nurse after ten years of service. She could have worked more years, but a Saudi Law expat working in a government hospital has an age limit of 60 years old only. She loved being a nurse; she was a devoted and dedicated nurse to all her patients. She advocated a patient-centered care approach to nursing on her staff to follow because she believes that nursing is a CARING profession. She also had a degree in education, but she pursued a nursing career as she found it more fulfilling and satisfying. Like the mother of nursing, Florence Nightingale, believed that nurses' presence with a patient is a key stone for making a professional communication. Empathy with patients and making an effort to relieve suffering and bringing them back to health she believed should be a mission of every nurse.

After retirement, she came back to the Philippines to focus more on her family and to do things that she enjoyed doing which she was not able to do when she was working. She was also a devout Roman Catholic, a devotee of "Sacred heart of Jesus", and "couple for

Christ" fellowship. Serving God faithfully was one of her greatest spiritual aspirations.

Things could not have been better for her - her daughter just got married and her son just finished school. She was also actively involved in her local church, so life is good for her.

Until one day, on October 20, 2019, she just finished showering when she was doing her own breast self-examination, which she normally does after shower, when she felt a mass the size of a kernel around 9 'o'clock position on her right breast. At first, she ignored thinking it was just a simple cyst because it's asymptomatic. However, a month later when she was on vacation in her hometown, she started to feel pain and also noticed redness around the area of the mass. Anxious and worried, she immediately went to the hospital to have it checked. She completed laboratories, Mammography and ultrasound on both breasts.

After two weeks of waiting like eternity the result of mammogram was confirmed:
- lobulated hypoechoic solid nodules;9-10 o'clock at the [r] breast biopsy recommended
- Birads category 4; [r] breast: suspicious abnormality, biopsy recommended
- Birad category 3; [l] breast, probably benign findings.

On December 4,2019, excision biopsy was done at the right mass breast. After two weeks the result confirmed that she had clusters of malignant ductal cells displaying enlarged round to pleomorphic, hyperchromatic nuclei, prominent nucleoli and scant cytoplasm with indistinct borders.

As a nurse with decades of experience she had an inkling idea what this means - she has cancer.

Upon learning the result of the biopsy, she felt nauseated, shocked and numb - she felt no emotion. She was afraid that she might die, I think is the common reaction of anyone being told that they have cancer. She was devastated, sad and depressed. She felt like her world was about to crumble into pieces. She couldn't sleep and eat - just thinking about her cancer and what it would do to her family. The only thing that makes her stronger and fights this cancer is her faith in God. She believes that God will help her overcome these trials in her life whatever path this cancer would take her.

"God unto thy hand I commend my life. Please, give me strength and courage so that I may be able to face whatever lies ahead. I am scared, but I will be strong in knowing that you will be by my side. As you promise that you will not give us a trial beyond what we can bear, but if you do, you will provide for us the way so that we may be able to endure it," she prayed to God.

She felt good after that prayer. She felt God's presence, rejuvenating her spirits; it made her relax and focus on the tasks ahead to think clearly about what's the best course of action and how to tell her family about her discovery that she had cancer. Right after she came home from her vacation, she told her family about her having been diagnosed with cancer. They were all devastated, and shocked, but extremely supported.

"We will get through this as a family. We are here for you, we will fight this cancer until we will defeat it," her husband and kids reassured her.

But things are not that easy, because to get this treatment you need the money. And they're not cheap! She didn't waste any time because as a nurse knew that time is of the essence - cancer does not lay dormant while she is looking for some ways to find a solution on how to get treatment. She called PGH [Philippines General Hospital], a government run hospital which gives a lot of free service to people that don't have the means. It's not that easy to get a check-up at PGH due to the queue of patients. However, things were running smoothly, she finished the required laboratories including HER2, ERA, and PRA. Unfortunately, there were no available slots for the admission for charity because a lot of other patients were waiting before her. She was given an option which was; If she wants urgent surgery immediately, she needs to go to a private hospital and pay for the surgery. She was told to prepare between 60-90 thousand pesos. She was distraught upon hearing it, as she knew her financial status. Her husband and her were both retired. The pension they are receiving is hardly enough to cover their monthly expenses, as both of them are on maintenance of high blood pressure and cholesterol pills. Her youngest son is working, but still on minimum wage and her daughter has her own family to look after, and the last thing she wants is to burden her with her own problems.
It was sometime in March; I saw her online when I glanced at who amongst our family members is online on messenger [we have a family group chat]. So, I said hello as I normally do whenever I saw anyone Online.

"Hello Manang! How are you doing these days?" I asked with enthusiasm.

"Not doing so well, Buds. I have been diagnosed with breast cancer," she said in a melancholic tune.

"Oh, I am so sorry to hear that Manang!" I said sadly.

That's when she opened up about her problem of not having the money to pay for the surgery if she opted to go to a private hospital. If she waits for the charity or "service patient" service she may be waiting for a long time as there are a lot of people ahead of her on the list. She does not have that time or the luxury to wait as time is of importance every passing moment. The earlier she gets the treatment the better chance of survival she is going to have. Without hesitation, I told her not to worry because we are going to pay for it - I am going to talk this over to my other cousin here in Canada. We were raised by our grandmother and our parents about the importance of family. My grandmother used to tell us;

"I don't care if you squabble, scream at each other, what I care about is that if your family needs you I expect you to march and be with your family. Because family is what defines us, without our family, then we are nothing!" told us like a broken record over and over.

After I hung up the phone, I called all my cousins in Canada to let them know about Manang Monin's predicament. Upon learning it, they all offered to pitch in to make up that amount. Right away, I message Manang Monin to go ahead and book the surgery as we will foot the bill for her surgery. My cousin was extremely grateful and ecstatic to hear the news. She went ahead and had herself admitted as a patient. Admission appointment with bed reservation was made and surgery is scheduled for March 3, 2020.

Unfortunately, bad luck or God is just testing her faith - how far she is going to continue trusting Him. It's easy to have faith when everything is going great. The real test of faith is when you're facing something that only your faith in God will get you through. On March 16,2020, another problem arose; all hospitals in the Philippines were closed due to covid-19 pandemic, which means her surgery that had been scheduled had to be canceled. She was extremely distraught upon learning it. She was stressed out, depressed, and had no appetite to eat. She is scared that the cancer cells might spread to other parts of her body. But as gloomy as it seemed her current situation, she still believed that God will provide the way for her to have surgery.

A good Samaritan from the couple of Christ family advised her to go to De La Salle Dasmarinas University Hospital. Thank God their outpatient department was open with limited patients per day. After four months of anxiously waiting, she started her OPD check-up at the De La Salle Dasmarinas University Hospital. All laboratories and diagnostic procedures were repeated. The result was satisfactory and she was cleared for surgery. However, since it was the peak of Covid of covid pandemic, her surgery was postponed three times.

Finally, she was admitted on August 8, 2020 in preparation for her surgery. On August 4, of the same year, at last she had her surgery and it was successful. She was discharged the next day. Post operation ultrasound was done - no sign of malignancy; all nodules are free. She was prescribed to take Tetrazole daily by her oncologist while waiting for her chemotherapy.

On November 5, 2020, her Adjuvant chemotherapy started with the following drugs as part of her treatment regimen: Cyclophosphamide and Doxorubicin every 3 weeks 4 cycles, Docetaxel every 3 weeks for 4 cycles and Trastuzumab every 3 weeks for 17 cycles. She was able to finish her 26 cycles of chemotherapy without severe side effects, except losing her hair. Letrozole drugs were stopped on June 1,2021, but restarted and she was advised to take it for the next five [5] years. On March 23, 2023, the oncologist added Zoledronic to be given via IV infusion every six months for the next five years.

Emotionally, psychologically and financially was an extremely difficult journey for her and her family, but God never abandoned her without help. What she had learned living with cancer, was that life is a journey, where each one of us have to travel the many twists and turns, highways and byways of life. We have to be strong, determined and unwavering in order for us to get to the other side. Moreover, we have to treasure every moment of our life with the people we love as we don't know what tomorrow may bring.

At present, she is coping well, going strong and am so grateful that she has a family who supported her through thick and thin - walked with her during those difficult journeys living with cancer. They were nothing but supported both emotionally and financially. Her heartfelt thanks to her children, husband, cousins, nieces, nephews, best friends and her Couples for Christ family. Last, but not the least, she would like to extend her gratitude to all government agencies and politicians such as, the Department of Health, PCSO [Philippines Charity Sweepstakes Office], DSWD

[Department of Social Welfare and Development], and others, who supported and get her free some of her treatment drugs from the beginning until the end of her treatment.

She is hoping and praying that this will continue until she can say to herself that *"I AM CANCER FREE!"*.

Tacing [describe in chapter 11]

She was a woman of faith, a philanthropist. She was diagnosed of Cervical cancer. After over a year of fighting valiantly, she unfortunately died and joined her creator where there is no more pain and suffering.

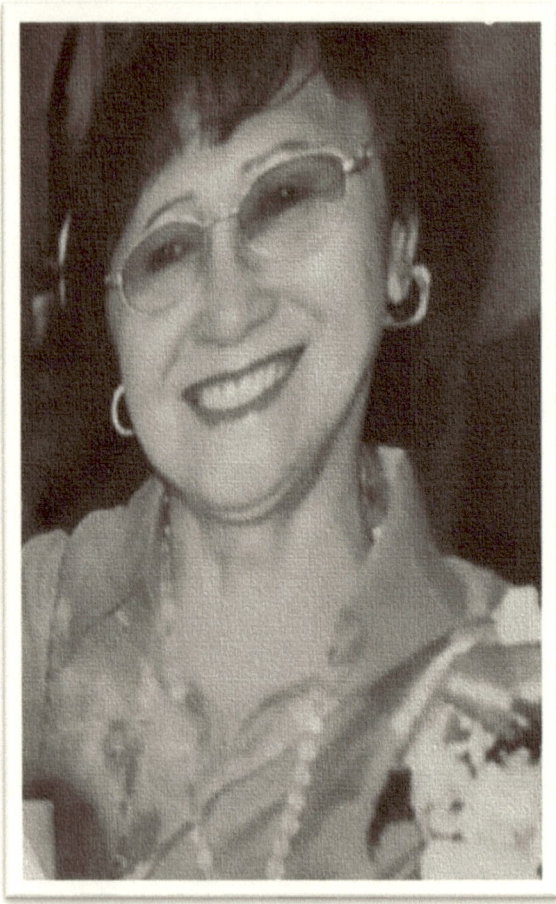

Chapter 11

A woman of faith

This is the story of Taciana Sta. Barbara de Otoy. She is a humble and truthful servant of God by living a life dedicated to serving the sick and the needy. Since childhood, her life had been marred with pain, financial difficulties, and suffering. This continued until she got married to her first husband and was employed in a public office. But her life with the Lord became different when she met her second husband [my nephew].

Taciana was born into a humble family whose daily income is derived from the sales of grocery items at her mother's neighborhood sundry store. As this income was only enough to help them stay alive, her elder sister, named Lydia Sta. Barbara Capistrano, had to stop studying and at a very young age, was forced to work as a laundry woman. With Lydia's hard labor, Taciana was able to study in a private school. For their family, quality education is a great equalizer since it could open the door to jobs, resources, and skills that may help them not only survive but thrive.

Taciana earned a Bachelor's Degree in Public Administration at the University of the Philippines and worked initially as a teacher in a government - owned learning institution, called Baclaran Elementary School. To build her career, she joined the National Cottage Industries Development Authority as a researcher and then worked at the Department of Trade and Industry [DTI] as chief of the International Services Division before she retired. At DTI, her hardship persisted as she fought a legal battle being a victim of the government reorganization. She was a pauper litigant with the Lord as the Lord as her lawyer, and through His love she won the case up to the Supreme Court. She also won eight other cases without a lawyer's prose in the face of the trial.

She was a devout Roman Catholic with an unshakable faith in God. The greenbelt Chapel became her sanctuary. For her, this was a place for refuge, protection, guidance, provision, security and justice with God. After office hours, she would visit the said chapel to praise God for the miracles performed and prayers answered. One afternoon, when the Blessed Sacrament was exposed, she saw the white Blessed Host turned into light pinkish orange. She shared this with a mass-goer, saying the Lord was giving her a message that she could not understand. The mass goer advised Taciana to visit the Christ the King Seminary and look for Grotto of the Annunciation for deeper contemplation. Following the advice, this marked the thirty-three [33] years of her journey in providing healing and deliverance service to the afflicted individuals.

After years when Taciana's first husband passed away, she met Aquilino de Otoy Jr. who was serving at the Sta. Rita de Casia Parish Church as a choir member. Taciana requested him to join her in serving the Lord at the said Grotto. Together, they then organized the Lord Jesus Christ the Living Word Ministry, which offered services such as healing, preaching, praying for the dead, and Life in the Spirit and Growth seminars at the Sta. Rita de Casia Parish Church. Widowed in 1990, Aquilino considered Taciana as a sister in the service of the Lord.

Taciana had undertaken, with Aquilino, several charitable activities. She supported financially deserving students to pursue their education as their families did not have the means to send their children to school. Gift packages containing rice, canned goods, and hygiene kits were provided annually to the elderly street dwellers every Easter Sunday and to indigent families on Christmas Day. She also mobilized her nephew, Doctor Mel Capistrano to organize medical missions and render free consultations and free medicines to the sick and poor individuals.

In 1997, when Aquilino fetched her from the international airport as she was coming home from her scholarship studies in Israel and visit to eleven [11] other countries, Aquilino frailness caught her attention. Taciana asked if Aquilino was sick. He said that he was fasting for fear that Taciana would not come back. It was then that Aquilino admitted missing her and had loved her since the day they had first met. Based on the advice of a priest, constant prayer, and discernment in the midst of tribulations, God consented to their marriage in 1999 at the St. Paul Church in Bergen, Norway.

It was Aquilino's great desire to serve God at the Greenbelt Chapel, as he wanted to become closer to God and to thank Him for His blessings. In response to the then chaplain, Rev. Fr. Anton CT Pascual's invitation, Aquilino joined the Healing Ministry and became one of the lay ministers.

On September 11,2021, they were schedule to attend the ISO community seminar the following day. My nephew, Aquilino, had a terrible cough so he decided to sleep in the other room as he didn't want Taciana to catch a cold from him. He didn't know that she fell and collapsed on the floor during the night. He found her lying on the floor when he woke up in the morning in a terrible shape. He attempted to get her up but she was so heavy for him and besides she was in extreme pain whenever he tried to lift her up. He went to get some help, but even then, they couldn't get her on her feet as she in excruciating pain. It was then that Aquilino had decided to call an ambulance as he didn't know the extent of her injury. It took six hours for the ambulance to come.

She was taken to St. Luke Medical Center in Manila, but prior for being taken in, you have to undergo a stringent Covid-19 protocol as it was the height of covid at the time. After two days the results came back and Taciana was positive for covid, and her husband Aquilino was also found positive three [3] days after. They were both quarantines. Unfortunately, the X-ray, and CT scan revealed that Taciana injured herself from the fall, resulting in severe compression deformity of her 12th thoracic vertebra and was admitted at St. Luke's Medical Center in September, 2021. However, the quarantine had adverse effects on Aquilino, as he had never been separated from Taciana since they were married. Aquilino, had some psychotic symptoms such as delirium, and delusion. Taciana was concerned for his well-being, so, she told the doctor who was in charge of her care that she wanted to go home.

"Mrs. de Otoy, you have a fracture, you need to stay in the hospital until you at least stand on your feet," the doctor advised her.

"I am going home with my husband. I will get a private Physiotherapist to help me get better. We will *quarantine at home. My husband's well being is my first priority at this moment, not my fracture,"* she strongly asserted to her doctor.

Against the medical advice of her doctor, she checked herself out of the hospital and went home with Aquilino. With her unshakable faith in God, she prayed for Aquilino's healing. After a few weeks, a miracle happened. Aquilino was slowly back to being himself again and Taciana's fracture was getting better through the help of a private physiotherapist that came to the house. They went back to their regular routine – serving God!

However, in June, Aquilino observed that she was always in the room, in bed and with no energy. What was alarming was that Aquilino became aware that Taciana's abdomen had grown big.

    "Are you okay, Love?" he asked with concern and with affection.

    "I don't know, Love, but I don't feel well. I have a lot of pain in my lower abdomen," she sadly uttered. Aquilino was worried that something could be seriously brewing inside, so he told Taciana that she was going to take her to the hospital. But before that, he asked their priest friend to come to the house to perform an anointing for the sick on her.

Taciana was admitted in the hospital to find out what was causing her abdomen to grow big and also to address other ailments and complaints such as difficulty in bowel movement [constipation]. After a series of blood work, further tests, CT Scan and MRI she was diagnosed with malignant cancer of the uterus. The cancer was already in the late stage – it had already metastasized and spread to the organs and cells. That explained why the abdomen had grown bigger because of ascites, excess fluid builds up in her peritoneal cavity. The oncologist who was treating her called for a meeting with immediate family: Aquilino, her son, her nephew [Dr. Mel Capistrano], and her cardiologist on what the course of action in terms of the treatment plan for her. It was suggested by the oncologist and in agreement by Taciana's nephew that she needed to have surgery – to remove the tumor and relieve her pain of the growing mass and ascites. Aquilino was devastated about Taciana's diagnosis. Just the thought of losing her brought anguish and shredding his hear into pieces.

Taciana was the love of his life, his mentor, and his strength and his joy. He could never love another woman, the way he had loved her despite their age gap. Taciana had accepted him for who he is. They were not just a husband and wife, but as well as they were best friends, confidant and partners in serving God.

"Lord, oh God! I pray for my beloved wife that you will heal her from this cancer and bring her back too health. Please, I am begging you to spare her life," Aquilino prayed earnestly to God.

The surgery had taken eight hour eight [8] hours, but it was successful. They were able to remove all the tumor – the surgical oncologist performed a radical hysterectomy [removal of the uterus, cervix, the upper part of the vagina, ovaries, fallopian tubes and nearby tissues]. After she got stronger, Aquilino took Taciana home to recuperate, although they were in and out of the hospital for the check - ups and follow ups.
Her last check-up, she was admitted again in the hospital because her oncologist noted something was

not right, after further blood tests and scan, it was revealed that her kidneys had failed – she therefore needed dialysis, and that was the beginning of her demise. Her vital organs started to shut down. Even the veins collapsed. It was very hard on Aquilino to watch his beloved wife suffer and nearing death. She affectionately asked him if he could lay beside her in bed and hold her in his arms. He did, with tears streaming down his cheeks, his heart broken because he knew that maybe this was going to be his last intimate moment with his darling and beloved wife.

"Love, when I am gone, I want you to continue your life and to continue serving the Lord. There is more than enough money for you to use to continue our advocacy – serving the less fortunate and doing the work that the Lord has entrusted us to do. I am sorry that you have to do it alone from now on but don't worry although I may not be with you physically but I will always be up there looking down on you. I will always be your prayer warriors. I love you Love, always and forever. From eternity and beyond." Taciana said, giving Aquilino her last wish.

"I love you too, Love. Thank you for loving me and accepting me for who I am. You are my greatest Love. My life will forever be better because you've been a part of it. I wish we could have more time together, but I want you to know that I will cherish the times we have had together. Thanks for being the one and only you and for being a blessing to so many people – especially me. I promise you that I will do what you asked me to do. I will continue to serve the Lord," Aquilino uttered in tears, holding Taciana so tight, afraid to let her go.

"Love, can I ask you one last request?" Looking Aquilino in the eye.

"Yes, Love. What is it?" he asked

"Would you mind washing me and making sure I am clean, including my private parts?" her voice was inaudible.

Despite two successive invasive operations to remove the cancer and treatments after a year of enduring the pain, side effects of treatments and coping with life living with cancer, on September 10, 2022 she succumbed to her death and joined her creator. She died peacefully. She accepted her fate from the bottom of her heart, never complained even once about her having cancer. She never faltered on her faith. She died happy and at peace because He believes that she served her purpose in life.

Aquilino did exactly as Taciana requested, almost blinded by the tears which were streaming down his face.

After he was finished washing Taciana, he called the pain management team in which he was instructed to do so, so that she would not suffer anymore. Then he called her son at 9 o'clock in the morning; he didn't come until 6 o'clock pm. At about 6:35 in the evening, Aquilino just turned his back toward the door as he wanted her son to have a private moment with his mother when she went *"flatline"*. He instructed them not to revive her anymore as that's her last wish.

Taciana was diagnosed with cancer in June/2022. Despite two successive invasive operations to remove the cancer and treatments after just a little more than three [3] months of enduring the pain, side effects and treatments and coping with life living with cancer. On September 10, 2022 she succumbed to her death and joined her creator. She died peacefully. She accepted her fate from the bottom of her heart, never complained even once about her having cancer. She never faltered in her faith. She died happy and at peace because she believed that she serves her purpose in life – serving the Lord.

It's hard on Aquilino to live a life without his beloved wife and his partner not only in marriage but as well as a partner in serving God. To keep his mind, occupied, he busied himself serving God and continued to do the work that his beloved wife started. Until today, Aquilino is still a lay minister even though he is involved with other ministers from other churches. He is continuously rendering service for the Glory of God at the Greenbelt Chapel as this was one of Taciana's requests before she died.

Aquilino always recalls the fondness they had together – as husband and wife. He also remembers in the remaining few days of his wife at the hospital, the struggle of offering her to God to end her suffering and the irony of wanting her to live and be with her forever. To be closer to her, he never failed to visit her gravesite and spend time with her. He believes that one day, he and Taciana will be reunited again. Cancer took away his beloved wife but, cancer cannot take away his love for her.

It's hard on Aquilino to live a life without her beloved wife and her partner not only in marriage but as well as a partner in serving God. To keep her mind occupied, he busied himself serving God and continued to do the work that his beloved wife started. Until today, Aquilino is still a lay minister even though he is involved with other ministers from other churches. He is continuously rendering service for the glory of God at the Greenbelt Chapel as this was one of Taciana 's requests before she died. Aquilino always recalls the fondness they had together with Taciana as husband and wife. He also remembers in the remaining few days of her wife at the hospital, the struggle of offering her to God to end her suffering and the irony of wanting her to live and be with her forever.

Chapter 12

Living with cancer and coping with the lost

Living with cancer

A cancer diagnosis can be an unexpected-life changing experience for patients and families. While learning about the diagnosis, you go through different experiences, various reactions such as shock, disbelief, confusion, sadness, anger, guilt, resignation, anxiety and depression. It can affect the emotional health of patients, families, and caregivers.

Speaking from experience, as a primary caregiver not just of one cancer patient but few of my family members. The first thing I vividly recalled the moment I heard the words:

"Sorry, your niece, your aunt, your sisters have cancer!" was a shock.

Death is the first thing that comes to mind; they are going to die. For a person who had been diagnosed with cancer and their family was devastating - you have to go through a whirlwind of emotions. It would take some time to sink in the reality that your loved one has cancer. Sometimes, it has to get worse before it gets better. From the moment of diagnosis, seeking treatment and the side effects of treatment was emotionally, mentally and physically overwhelming.

Just as cancer affects your physical health, it can also bring a wide range of emotions you're not used to dealing with. It can also make an existing feeling seem more intense. They may change daily, hourly, or even moment by moment. This is true whether you're currently in treatment, done with the treatment, or a friend or family member. I was a primary caregiver of four people who were extremely close to me that had been diagnosed with cancer, except my sister as she lived in the Philippines. However, I was involved in my sister's treatment and care until she succumbed to her death. Each one of them had different types of cancer: my niece [Acute Myelogenous Leukemia], my adopted mother [Ovarian cancer], my adopted sister [breast cancer], her sister [colon cancer], and last year my older sister [Laryngeal or throat cancer]. Each one of them had different reactions, and feelings in accepting the fact that they had been diagnosed with cancer. Some accepted it quickly; others took them sometimes to accept. There is no right or wrong in the way you react to your diagnosis of having cancer. These feelings are all normal. You are entitled to express how you feel. Often the values you grew up with will affect how you think about and cope with cancer. For me, I need to be strong to protect my family and friends. But what really helps me get through and cope during those difficult times is my faith in God. Whatever you decide, it's important to do what's right for you and not compare yourself with others. Your friends and family members may share some of the same feelings.

As I had mentioned in the previous chapter of this book, my first encounter with cancer was when my thirteen years old niece was diagnosed with Acute Myelogenous Leukemia [AML], less than two months after she was diagnosed she passed away. I was her primary caregiver as her mother was working in Hong Kong, as an Overseas Foreign Worker or [OFW]. At a young age, I watched how cancer slowly destroyed my young niece's body. I watched her groan in pain day and night. I watched her slowly wither away – fade slowly in front of my eye. I could think of a fully vibrant grown leaf that starts off green, and then slowly changes color before it falls off the tree. Then when it lands it starts to decompose, before it gets absorbed into the ground and disappears. At a young age, I didn't understand why she had to die of cancer. She was just a kid. It took me sometimes to get over her death, especially what she endured during those horrible times.

Cancer diagnosis is overwhelming to the patients and to the family, especially if you are a primary caregiver. The moment you've learned that your loved one had cancer, you feel as if your life is spiraling out of control. Sadness starts to crawl in because you wonder if they are going to die. Your normal routine is disrupted by doctors' visits and treatment. You feel like you can't do a lot of things you enjoyed before, and you feel helpless and lonely.

Anger

Anger was one of the first reactions of someone who had been diagnosed with cancer. It's very normal to ask "why me?" or "why my loved ones?" and be angry at the cancer. You may also feel anger or resentment towards your health care providers, your healthy friends and your loved ones. And if you are religious, you may even feel angry with God.

I remembered, My adopted sister when she was first diagnosed with cancer, she was hysterical! She was

193

crying uncontrollably and so angry with herself for neglecting the previous advice of her doctor to have her breast checked regularly because she had papilloma removed a few years back, but she had ignored the advice of the doctor who performed the surgery. I just stood there, holding her hands but I did not stop her because sometimes it helps to get that anger out of your system. I just told her that what's done cannot be undone. What we should be focusing and spending our energy is on how to deal with the situation – her cancer.

You feel angry, it's okay, you don't have to pretend that you're okay when you're not. It's not healthy to keep it inside you. Sometimes anger can be helpful in a short term, for it motivates you to take action. However, having constant anger or resentment won't feel good to you or the people around you. But each one of us has different ways of "coping mechanism" on how we deal or cope with a stressful thing in our life. Change is constant, and when it happens, it can feel overwhelming. That's true whether the change is positive or negative, expected or unexpected. When this happens, we look for ways to cope with a stressor while trying to keep our emotional balance. Coping mechanisms are the patterns and behaviors we fall back on to try to deal with unusually stressful situations – like cancer. We often lean on these strategies to keep ourselves calm until we adjust to the change or stressful time. Imagine that you are stepping onto a boat. When you put your foot on the deck, you feel the boat start to move beneath you. You hold on tightly to the shroud until you get your footing. A short while later, you're standing and talking to a friend on the boat when it suddenly begins to move. You stumble, looking for support behind you. the movements of the boat are your changing circumstances. Your instincts to reach out for support are your coping mechanisms. And, as any sailor will tell you, certain parts of the boat are better to hold on to than others.

What helps me, even though I feel things are out of control, I focus on the things I still have control over and find ways to take charge of some things. I do a lot of reading and learn as much as I can about the many types of cancer, its characteristics, and treatments to help me and my loved one diagnosed with cancer navigate through it. The more knowledge I have, the more in control I'll feel. What I found helpful, before our doctor appointment I would prepare a list of questions to ask the doctor and the rest of the health team involved in my loved one's care and to say, "explained to me" if there are things not clear and I don't understand. I believe that patients and family members are within their boundaries to ask questions and be objective, after all, it is you or your loved one's life that we are talking about.

Fear and worry

It's scary to hear that you or your loved one have cancer. Because of traumatic experiences I had with my niece when she was diagnosed with Acute Myelogenous Leukemia – she suffered terribly and eventually died less than two months after she was diagnosed. I therefore associated cancer to death and suffering. I was afraid and terrified that like my niece, I will lose them too. I was worried about them being in pain, either from cancer or treatment. I worry about them feeling sick or worry about the side effects of treatment. How would I take care of them, and keep my job at the same time? Is not easy because not all employers are supported and understanding. At one time I was told either to come to work or lose my job. I was livid and hurt at the same time, but abandoning my loved one who is fighting for their life is never an option.

"If you want to fire me, that's your prerogative. However, just make sure you fire me for the right reason, not because I am tending to my family who is fighting for her life." I firmly asserted this to my manager.

You get stressed out from the barrage of questions every time you take a day off to accompany your loved one to her treatment or doctor's appointment. You thought to yourself, "maybe just take a leave of absence", but then you worry about where to get the money to pay the bills [household expenses], and others.

Although some fear about cancer is based on stories, rumors, or wrong information. I found to cope with fears and worries it often helps to be well informed. Most people feel better when they learn the fact. They feel less afraid when know what to expect. Learning about your cancer and understanding what you can do to be an active partner in your care helps base in my experience.

Sad and depressions

Sadness is a normal reaction of many people diagnosed with cancer. They feel the sense of loss of their health, and the life they had before they learned they had cancer. I remember Nana, Lita and Neneng; how extremely sad they were when they found out they had the disease. Even when they are done with the treatment, they still feel sad. I think this is a common response to any serious illness. It took them some time to walk through and accept that they have cancer and all the changes that are taking place.

When you're sad, you may have very little energy, feel tired or no appetite to eat. For some, these feelings go away or lessen over time. but for others, these emotions can become stronger as they journey through living with cancer. The painful feelings don't get any better, and they get in the way of daily life. This sadness sometimes falls into depression. All of my family members who were diagnosed with cancer went through this emotional mood disorder. But as much as it's hard on them it's also extremely hard on the people who care for them, especially for the primary caregiver. You have to keep fighting for them, be strong not just for them but for yourself too. Because you can't afford to fall apart especially if you're the only one that they have to rely on to care for them. You have to deal with their mood swing, resentment and other negative feelings. You have to keep assuring and reiterating to them that you love them and they will not go through with it alone.

Guilt

If you feel guilty, know that many people with cancer feel this way. They feel guilty for upsetting the people they love and feel that they are a burden to them. Nana and Lita used to feel guilty for getting me into trouble at work. My sister, Neneng Herminia, feels guilty for spending my hard-earned money for her treatment.

Some people feel envious when they see other people in good health and are ashamed of this feeling afterwards. Sometimes, they might even blame themselves for their lifestyles, choices that they think could have led to their getting cancer. But as I always said to my loved one;

"Getting cancer is never your fault! There are a lot of things that are beyond our control, and one of them is getting sick of cancer."

Financial

I didn't realize how lucky I am to be living here in Canada until I was confronted with my sister's cancer diagnosis. In Canada, we complain about every little thing; like waiting at the emergency and waiting at the doctor's office - we are spoiled in a lot of ways. We bad mouth the system! What we don't realize is what other people had to go through to get helped, especially those diagnosed with cancer.

When Nana, Lita, and Libeth were diagnosed with cancer, I never had to worry about where I was going to get the money to pay for their treatment. Everything has been done and arranged by the doctor and the health team. If you don't have private insurance at work, the trillium insurance in partnership with OHIP [Ontario Health Insurance], or other provincial health insurance pays for your treatment. Not only that, the doctors, social workers and other health teams provide all the support needed to make it easier for you to navigate as you journey through life living with cancer. They also provide homecare services [palliative doctors, nurses, and PSW] to come to the house to care for the patients and make it easier for the primary caregiver to cope. They also provide equipment's [hospital bed, oxygen, mechanical lift and other medical supplies] to give the patients more comfort whilst staying in the home. However, when my sister in the Philippines was diagnosed with cancer, I was confronted with the grim reality which I am not used to. We have to pay for everything [doctors, laboratories, scan and other imaging, treatment and caregiver, oxygen, suction machine and other medical supplies]. I can't just imagine what it's like for those people that don't have the means. Like in the case of Alberto and Nelly Lorea's son, Neil Albert Lorea, a seventeenth years old young man who was diagnosed of Diffuse B-Cell Lymphoma or [DBCL], who died four months later after he was diagnosed [he was described in one of the chapters of this book]. I heard the excruciating pain expressed by Neil's parents of not having the means to provide for their son's treatment when I went to interview them in the Philippines. According to them it's bad enough that their son had cancer, but to lack the means of giving him a chance to survive was even worse. Yes, the government of the Philippines have agency, like PhilHealth [insurance given by the government], Department of Social Welfare and Development [DSWD], and Local Government Unit [LGU] – who help and assist the needs of those underprivileged or downtrodden gets help they needed and *"service patient"* who gets free doctor and hospital but still have to pay for the treatment, imaging and laboratories even if its discounted. The other problem which existed according to reliable sources [*anonymous], is that most of the time the people who benefited from the government program were those well off and have connections, not really the downtrodden. They abused the system; by using their connection to get free medical services. Henceforth, by the time it gets to the people who really need it the money allocated to the program has already been exhausted.

The doctor – Patient Relationship

The doctor has an integral role in your cancer diagnosis because you rely on your doctor to give you clear and helpful information that will guide you through making decisions about your care. Your doctor relies on you to be open and honest, and to trust them. Yes, trust is very important in a doctor-patient relationship. You need to be able to trust your doctor that he/she will act in your best interest. In this way, you and your doctor are collaborators – a team working together to make sure you get the best care possible. Remember everyone is different. It can take time to plan and make treatment decisions when you have cancer. There are many factors to consider, based on my experience when my loved ones were diagnosed with cancer, it's important to learn all you can about cancer. But, it's also important to remember that each person's cancer experience is different. There are many different types of cancer and subtypes of tumors that make a person's experience and treatment options different from someone else's. There are also other non-cancer health problems and factors that can affect how cancer and treatment might be planned and given. However, while there are many resources for information, your first and foremost resource should be your doctor and others who are part of your cancer care team because they know your situation best. Talking to your doctor isn't always easy, but it's important to remember that your doctor is often the only person who can answer certain questions, not Mr. goggles!

Taking an active role is very important. Being a partner in your or your loved ones' cancer treatment can help you get the best care from the team of doctors, nurses and other health care providers taking care of you. It is also very important to discuss your concerns about how cancer will affect your life and the things you do. Don't be ashamed or shy about asking questions. There's no such thing as a *"dumb"* question. Simple rule, *"if you don't ask, you don't get an answer"*.

Getting a second opinion is very important. When Nana was diagnosed with Ovarian cancer, she was just given 2-4 months to live and sent home as a palliative care patient [comfort measure only]. However, after pondering and contemplating over it for a few days, I talked to Nana's general Practitioner [GP] and told him that I would like to seek a second opinion for my peace of mind. The *"what if?"* was kept playing in my mind like a broken record. Our GP or family doctor was very supportive – he always respects my opinion. He referred Nana to another Oncologist, and because of that Nana had lived for another three years. I still remembered what that second Oncologist said, *"my job as a doctor is to do my best to help my patient to live, not to tell them how long they have to live. That's the big Guy upstairs job, not mine."* Indeed! Getting a second opinion can help you feel sure about your or your loved ones diagnosis and treatment plan. The way I see getting a second opinion – you have nothing to lose but gain!

Simple act of kindness from the doctor and other health care team can help to diffuse negative emotions, based on my experience. Accurate diagnosis and treatment are paramount, of course, but how the care team delivers care also matters, as it can be a potent antidote to patients' and family's negative emotions and may improve their outcome. Empathy can also help create a safe space so that patients feel more comfortable sharing their experiences with their doctors and other health care teams. In my experience in dealing with doctors and other health care teams, I was blessed because my loved ones who had been diagnosed with cancer had excellent doctors and health care providers. Special mention to my sister's doctors and health care team in the Philippines, who had been nothing but supportive and understanding, specially Doctor Rosalinda Palmares who had been exemplary; always went out of her way to help my sister and helped me coped on how to navigate my sister's cancer diagnosis and likewise to my sister's Oncologist, Doctor A, whom like Doctora Palmares had been nothing but supportive, the same thing goes to my sister's radiologist/oncologist, Doctor D.

Thus, we associate compassion with an active desire to alleviate the suffering of its object, in the face of others. With sympathy, I feel for your hardship. With empathy, I share your emotions. With compassion, I can share your suffering and elevate it into a universal *"common humanity"* and transcending experience.

Surviving cancer

They said cancer is a journey that you have to walk through every day even if you survive it. Lita, thank goodness, has been cancer free for eleven years now, but sometimes there is always this fear and worry of recurrence. Living with uncertainty or *"fear of the unknown"* is the most difficult one. I always remind Lita that fear and anxiety are normal parts of survivorship. Worrying about cancer coming back is usually intense the first year after treatment, then it's gotten better every year. Some people reject the term survivor as being a narrow conceptualization of highly variable human experiences. It prefers to use the *"alivers"* and the *"thrivers",* which put emphasis on living as well as possible despite the fear and worry of cancer recurrence. I always told Lita that, *"cancer doesn't have to define you, instead you should define yourself".* And it is possible not just to survive cancer, but to thrive and live a healthy and happy life again, with a semblance of normalcy regardless of the scar cancer has left on your body, especially your life.. Just enjoy every day without worrying about tomorrow. As the saying goes, *"Life is 10% what happens to us and 90% how we react to it."* According to Epictetus, stoic Philosopher," We *should not moor a ship with one anchor, or our life with one hope."* The essence of this philosophy is that a man should live that his happiness shall depend as little as possible on external things. It is not death or pain that is to be dreaded, but the fear of pain and death.

Gratitude or living life every moment

What I had learned throughout my experience caring for my loved ones who had cancer I see their cancer as a *"wake up call".* I realized the importance of enjoying the little things in life. A lot of things in life that we have no control over, and one of them is what lies ahead and getting sick with cancer. However, we can control how we choose to live our life. We should try to be happy and appreciate every little thing we have and nurture them. Life is fragile, it can be taken away from us in a blink of an eye. According to Eckhart Tolle, *"When you go deeply into the present, gratitude arises spontaneously, even if it's just gratitude for breathing, gratitude for being alive that you feel in your body. Gratitude is there when you acknowledge the aliveness of the present moment; that's the foundation for successful living."*

A lot of things we wanted to do, more often we put aside, either by our busy schedules, or for some other reasons. I remembered, one of my client sons asked me,

"Loretta, have you been to Israel?" he asked.

"Not yet! But I plan to go there when I retire," I replied.

"Loretta, you should go places that you want to go while you are still able and strong. Don't wait for your retirement – the way you look it seems like retirement still a few years down the road. Who knows what will happened then?" He honestly remarks.

Thinking about it, he was absolutely right! Nana and my sister died of cancer and Lita was diagnosed, but survived after a long and difficult journey, it changed the way I see life. That life is fragile, we have no control over what happened to us the next day. We may be here today, but we could be gone tomorrow. We should cherish every moment while we are still alive and spend more time with the people we love – family and friends. We should mend a broken relationship. I am glad that I was able to make it right with my sister before she passed away. WE should also let the people we love know how much we value them. The other thing that I learned through this experience is that no matter how difficult things are, we should always try to look for the joy in life even though you have been diagnosed with cancer. Pay attention to the things you do each day that make you smile. They can be as simple as drinking your favorite coffee, spending quality time with your family, walking with friends or appreciating the beauty of nature. Whatever you choose, embrace the things that bring you joy when you can. As Lita said, *"I was given a second chance at life. I will darn enjoy it."* Indeed!

Gratitude is often quoted as being a core practice to a wholesome and fulfilling life. I am owed anything; we have been given the opportunity, to experience life, to create, to think, to build relationships. There are many people who have less than I have, and suffered more than I did, so therefore, I have so much to be grateful about. Gratitude is a process, a way of being mindful and opening up awareness to our surroundings, to past, present, and future events and to our experiences whether they be physical, mental, emotional, and cognitive. In a nutshell, to me gratitude can simply the importance of seeing the positives no matter how bad is your situation

Coping with the lost

If nothing else, death is a constant reminder of the fragility of life. It is a reminder of our existence and the time we have. Through death, we are reminded of why life is so valuable. But the hardest pill to swallow is that we, like everything else in life, must pass.

This is an abstract concept, where one moment we are alive and then in the blink of an eye we're not. There is no escape, no avoidance, no prevention. Each one of us we reach our expiry date; we will die. And on the face of it, that is extremely bleak. It leads some to live a hedonistic lifestyle while others turn to existential nihilism, asking what is the point in anything if we're just going to die? But we must accept that death is part of natural order. *"Death, like birth, is just a natural process, material elements combining, growing, decaying and finally separating and completely dispersing."* According to Marcus Aurelius.

I am no stranger to death, as I was exposed to death at a very young age when I was a primary caregiver to my 13 years old niece who had died of cancer less than two months after she had been diagnosed of Acute Myelogenous Leukemia, then more to followed after that: my three brothers of violence death, I lost my mother at the age of 57, my brother from a freak accident, my two nephews from a brutal and heinous death, not to mention my other two half siblings from natural death. Then, Nana, and recently my older sister, Neneng Herminia from Laryngeal cancer. So, I have more than a fair share when it comes to the death of loved ones. And I will tell you that coping with the loss of loved ones was very difficult to handle. Mourning is a process or journey that affects everyone differently. It can be exhausting and emotionally draining. Grief has no set pattern. It is expressed differently across different cultures. Some people like to be expressive and public with their emotions, while others like to keep it private. Most people lessen with time. A person who loses a loved one may always carry sadness and miss the person who had died, but they are able to find meaning and experience pleasure again. Some people even find new wisdom and strength after experiences of loss. There is no right or wrong when it comes to mourning or expressing your grief. Every death affects you differently: death of siblings, parents, spouses, friends and other people close to you. Some people are stronger than others and therefore, they coped better, while others were not strong enough to cope with the loss and it would take them longer to accept and get used to the idea that their loved ones were no longer around. Grief is a person's response to the loss of someone or something that was important to them. Grief can occur after death, divorce, illness or other significant loss. Grief can affect your mental and physical health. The experience of grief is different for everyone.

These losses aren't just felt at one time in a person's life; true the grief – form, they pop up as a milestone reminder: birthdays, important events, holidays and emptiness forever. I think the magnitude of this can be hard to recognize when looking at it from the outside in and I think those who experience the losses are often surprised by how hard "*acceptance*" is. When you care deeply about the person it can be difficult to know when to let go.

The hardest part about death is the physical separation; that the person you care so much and love were no longer around. You can't hear their voice talking back at you, nor do you see them smile again and you miss those times you regularly did with them.

I remembered my first vacation in the Philippines after my mother died. I didn't realize how much it hit me when I disembarked on the plane and came out of the airport without seeing my mother. In the past, her face was the first person I saw to welcome me back home whenever I came home for holiday. But now, she was no longer there among the crowd. It took me sometimes to get used to the idea that she was really gone. When Nana Carling died, it took me sometimes to get used to not having to see her when I come home from work and the first person I see when I wake up in the morning. When Neneng Herminia was diagnosed with cancer, to boost her spirit and to let her know that I am with her in her journey; I called her every morning when she wakes up and every evening before she goes to bed. After she died, sometimes, I still attempted to dial her phone, but stopped when realizing that she was not there anymore.

Her family:

"Miniang, It's hard for me to live a life without you – after forty-four [44] years of marriage. But I would try my best to move on for the sake of our grandchildren. I love so much! Until we meet again my beloved wife." Papa

"Mama, until now we can't accept that you left us already. But we love you so much, enough to let you go. Every time we see you gasping for air to breathe, or writing on a piece of paper to express what you wanted to say, it tears our heart – cut like a knife. Our only comfort was that you're not suffering anymore – no more pain! Thank you for being a good mother and extraordinary grandmother for your grandchildren. You will be forever in our heart. We love you and miss you so much!" Jonelle and Rochelle

"Mama, until now I still can't accept that you were no longer with us. I still see you in every corner of our house, hear your voice. Cancer robbed us with the most important person in our lives. But we have to accept it no matter how painful it is. I promise you that I would strive to finish my studies that you would be proud of me there in heaven looking down. I will become a nurse – like you! You are my mentor, my beloved Mama. I love you so much!" Moira Cassandra [MC]

"Mama, I am lost without you! Why do you have to die? I hate cancer for taking you away from me. I missed you so much! I am praying to God that He would let me see you again, even just in my dreams. I love you Mama!" UK

"I love you Mama!" Jayden

Nelly and Alberto Lorea when I interviewed them, I had to stop because they were so overwhelmed with sadness when I was asking them questions about their son. Brought them back to that horrible and painful experience of losing their only son to cancer.

Gerry my nephew, his way to cope with his loss is by visiting his beloved wife in her graveside - spending his whole day with her and by continuing doing what his wife asked him to do - continuing her charity brings him closer to her.

Death is probably the most challenging thing humans can face. It breaks us down. It brings us to our knees. Some people are so significant in our lives that the mere thought of living without them feels incredibly overwhelming and incapacitating. However, as hard as it may be, we have to accept that they're gone – no longer around. Acceptance helps us to cultivate inner peace, even amidst the unpredictability and challenges that are an inherent part of the human experience and most importantly, it helps us to move on. Getting used to the idea that they're no longer around. Accepting death of a loved one doesn't mean that we are forgetting about them, what it means is you are moving forward with life without them. But you still cherish that memory you had with them in your heart forever.

Flashbacks and Traumatic memories

Losing a loved one in any context is traumatic but losing someone to cancer often involves a number of traumatic experiences from diagnosis to treatment to palliative care. You may find that since your loved one passed away certain memories intrude into your mind without you choosing to think about it. Especially if you are a primary caregiver; you have witnessed all the suffering that your loved one had endured during their journey living with cancer. You stood their helpless – you want to help to ease their suffering but there is nothing that you can do to help, and that is the most excruciating and can be incredibly traumatic anyone could experience. You prayed to God to end the suffering and just take them away. This can be very distressing because these memories are often very painful to think about. However, we have no choice, but to accept that they are gone now. If any consolation for us; who loved them – they were no longer suffering.

Epictetus advises us to approach each situation with a sense of curiosity and adaptability. He encourages us to see setbacks and challenges as opportunities for growth and learning, rather than as obstacles to be feared or resisted. By doing so, we can cultivate an inner resilience that would help us navigate life's twists and turns with grace and equanimity.

Grief is like the ocean; it comes on waves ebbing and flowing. Sometimes the water is calm, and sometimes it is overwhelming. All we can do is learn how to swim, otherwise we will drown.

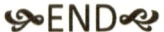 END

References:

All medical terms used in this book are taken from:
American Cancer Society, Canadian Cancer Society,
PSW text book, googles, Mayo Clinic and Wikipedia

www.ingramcontent.com/pod-product-compliance
Lightning Source LLC
Chambersburg PA
CBHW050442290526
45786CB00006B/2128